Gaffor Sadiq Omer

Diagnosing Aortic Valve Stenosis using Echocardiography Technique

Gaffor Sadiq Omer

Diagnosing Aortic Valve Stenosis using Echocardiography Technique

LAP LAMBERT Academic Publishing

Impressum / Imprint

Bibliografische Information der Deutschen Nationalbibliothek: Die Deutsche Nationalbibliothek verzeichnet diese Publikation in der Deutschen Nationalbibliografie; detaillierte bibliografische Daten sind im Internet über http://dnb.d-nb.de abrufbar.
Alle in diesem Buch genannten Marken und Produktnamen unterliegen warenzeichen-, marken- oder patentrechtlichem Schutz bzw. sind Warenzeichen oder eingetragene Warenzeichen der jeweiligen Inhaber. Die Wiedergabe von Marken, Produktnamen, Gebrauchsnamen, Handelsnamen, Warenbezeichnungen u.s.w. in diesem Werk berechtigt auch ohne besondere Kennzeichnung nicht zu der Annahme, dass solche Namen im Sinne der Warenzeichen- und Markenschutzgesetzgebung als frei zu betrachten wären und daher von jedermann benutzt werden dürften.

Bibliographic information published by the Deutsche Nationalbibliothek: The Deutsche Nationalbibliothek lists this publication in the Deutsche Nationalbibliografie; detailed bibliographic data are available in the Internet at http://dnb.d-nb.de.
Any brand names and product names mentioned in this book are subject to trademark, brand or patent protection and are trademarks or registered trademarks of their respective holders. The use of brand names, product names, common names, trade names, product descriptions etc. even without a particular marking in this works is in no way to be construed to mean that such names may be regarded as unrestricted in respect of trademark and brand protection legislation and could thus be used by anyone.

Coverbild / Cover image: www.ingimage.com

Verlag / Publisher:
LAP LAMBERT Academic Publishing
ist ein Imprint der / is a trademark of
OmniScriptum GmbH & Co. KG
Heinrich-Böcking-Str. 6-8, 66121 Saarbrücken, Deutschland / Germany
Email: info@lap-publishing.com

Herstellung: siehe letzte Seite /
Printed at: see last page
ISBN: 978-3-8465-8281-7

Zugl. / Approved by: University of Bolton, October 2012

LIST OF CONTENT: SUBJECTS PAGES

ACKNOWLEDGMENTS:

I would like to say thanks, to the Centre for Materials Research and Innovation (CMRI), University of Bolton staffs, especially my supervisor Prof. Martin Grootveld, Dr Tahir Shah, Dr Subbiyan Rajendran, Dr Mohsen Miraftab, Prof. Jack Lue, Prof. Anand and other staff and teachers. Also, many thanks to Preston Cardiac Respiratory staff, especially Mr Shahid Tagari, the manager of Cardio-Respiratory Departments at Preston and Chorley Hospital. Last but not least I would like to many thanks to my wife (Mhabat), she helped and supported me during studding my master, I much appreciate this indeed.

ABSTRACT:

Aortic stenosis (AS) is the most common valve disease in the West. It results in significant left ventricular (LV) changes, including myocardial hypertrophy, systolic and diastolic dysfunction. Aortic valve replacement (AVR) remains the only available management for AS and results in improved symptoms and recovery of ventricular function. However, it carries potential risks. In high-risk AS patients, such as the elderly or patients with severe LV dysfunction, the surgical risk could mount up to 3-4 folds, compared to that of younger patients or those with maintaining ventricular function and that rate progression and symptoms of Aortic Valve Stenosis. This study summarizes the current procedures and the emerging application of echocardiographic techniques in the diagnosis and management of asymptomatic severe aortic stenosis. Doppler echocardiography enables measurements of maximum aortic jet velocity, mean pressure aortic valve gradient and the aortic valve area by continuity calculation. The data measurements were collected from 215 patients within three different groups of aortic valve patients (Native Aortic Valves, Tissue Prosthetic Aortic Valve and Mechanical Prosthetic Aortic Valves). The subjects selected were from the years 2000 - 2012, who were suffering from Aortic Valve Stinosis. There were between 3 years and 11 years of measurement data available for each patient depending on the severity and symptomatic progression and correlation of underlying causes.

Data acquired was subjected to discriminatory analysis using maximum velocity, maximum gradient, mean gradient, LVF/EF, age, and total cholesterol, HDL-cholesterol, LDL-cholesterol and triacylglycerol levels as quantitative explanatory, active variables, and gender, rhythm status, renal function status, and category as qualitative explanatory variables (monitoring year was obviously excluded since this is a non-contributory variable). The participants were recruited from the Cardio-respiratory Department, Lancashire Teaching Hospital NHS Trust (Preston), United Kingdom. A step-by-step approach will be incorporated into the test. The measurements will be recorded before and after performing all tests within each subject, then the results will be compared within the subjects and between subject groups. The result shows there are a significant correlation between several acquired data measurements, including, age, maximum velocity, maximum gradient and mean gradients. Also, it shows that a great discrimination by a group of Tissue Prosthetic Aortic Valve (TPAV) compared to each of the Native Aortic Valves (NAV) group and Mechanical Prosthetic Aortic Valve (MPAV) groups.

LIST OF TABLES   **Page**

LIST OF FIGURES: **Page**

LIST OF WORD ABBREVIATIONS

ABBREVIATION	DETAILS
AR	Aortic regurgitation
AS	Aortic stenosis
AV	Aortic valve
BAV	Bicuspid aortic valve
CABG	Coronary Arterial Bypass Graft
CHD	coronary heart disease
CHF	Congestive heart failure
CVD	Cardiovascular disease
CVS	Cardiovascular system
EEG	Electroencephalogram
MI	Myocardial Infarction (heart attack)
MRI	Magnetic Resonance Imaging
AVR	Aortic Valve Replacement
TAVI	Trans-catheter aortic valve implantation
LA	Left Atrium
LV	Left Ventricle
RA	Right Atrium
RV	Right Ventricle
EF	Ejection fraction
LVOT	Left Ventricular Aortic Tract
2D-Echo	2Dimensional View Echocardiography
3D-Echo	3Dimensional View Echocardiography
CHD	Coronary Heart Disease
CAD	Coronary Artery Disease
CRD	Cardio Respiratory Department
HF	Heart Failure
ΔP	pressure gradient
SPSS	Statistical Package for the Social Sciences
ANOVA	Analyse Of Variation
LAE	Left Atrial Enlargement
NYHA	New York Heart Association

ΔP..pressure gradient

NSR..Normal Sinus Rhythm

AF..Atrial Fibrillation

SV..stroke volume

SVI..stroke volume index

LVOT ....left ventricular outflow tract

EDV...end diastolic volume

ESV..end systolic volume

SBP ....systolic blood pressure

CHAPTER

ONE

INTRODUCTION

1.0 INTRODUCTION:

Cardiovascular disease (CVD) is the major cause of death worldwide. Underlying causes, such as atherosclerosis and hypertension, are associated with remodelling of the vessel wall ultimately leading to loss of structural integrity. There are a number of factors that can influence vascular remodelling and hence structural integrity. The overall aim of this thesis was to investigate aortic wall integrity in relation to genetics and blood flow (Jacob D P, et al., 2008).

Aortic stenosis (AS) is the most common, valve disease in the West, with a prevalence varying between 0.02% in adults under 44 years and 3-9% in those over 80 years of age (Nkomo VT, et al., 2006, Iung B, et al., 2007). Aortic stenosis (AS) is an abnormal narrowing of the aortic valve. This narrowing restricts blood flow through the aortic valve into the aorta. The disease may remain silent "asymptomatic" and hence unnoticed for years, particularly in the elderly, with naturally limited exercise. The more narrowed the valve, the less blood can go through AV, the more severe the symptoms and problems are likely. Severe AS can cause symptoms and may lead to heart failure. A normal aortic valve area (AVA) is 3-5 cm^2, if the AVA is less than 0.8 cm^2, then severe AS is likely. With the development of symptoms, patients may carry a mortality of 36-52%, 52-80% and 80-90% in 3, 5 and 10 years, respectively if left untreated, even carrying a high risk of sudden death (Rajamannan NM, et al., 2008). Aortic valve replacement (AVR) is the only effective treatment for severe AS; it is indeed the second indication for open heart surgery after coronary artery bypass grafting (CABG) (Bridgewater B, et al., 2011).

The condition of AS, appear more in men than women, with a ratio of 3:1. AS, is considered to be the third most common cardiovascular disease, after hypertension and coronary artery disease respectively. There are several techniques that can diagnose AS, these include; Electrocardiography (ECG), X-ray, Cardiac Catheterisation, Echocardiography and Microwave Radiometry (MR). This project is about diagnosing AS and we are using the Echocardiography technique during the test trail project. The trial is based on NHS Trust hospital and all patients are recruited from Preston and Chorley Cardiac Respiratory Department (Busko M, 2011).

Native Aortic Valve Stenosis:

Calcification of native tricuspid and congenital bicuspid valves is the most common cause of aortic stenosis in industrialized countries (figure 1). There is compelling evidence that thickening and calcification in aortic valve disease is a complex inflammatory process and not simply age-related degeneration. Both aortic sclerosis and stenosis represent phenotypic expressions of one disease continuum. Patients with symptomatic severe aortic stenosis benefit from aortic valve replacement. However, management in the absence of symptoms remains challenging. While a delay of aortic valve replacement due to lack of symptom recognition may result in a dismal outcome, unselected premature aortic valve replacement may be associated with unbalanced risks of cardiac surgery. Echocardiography is the standard for evaluating the severity of aortic stenosis; however, most of the current echocardiographic parameters have limitations in predicting the onset of symptoms (figure 2). This review summarizes the current guidelines and the emerging application of echocardiographic techniques in the diagnosis and management of asymptomatic severe aortic stenosis (Jacob D P, et al., 2008).

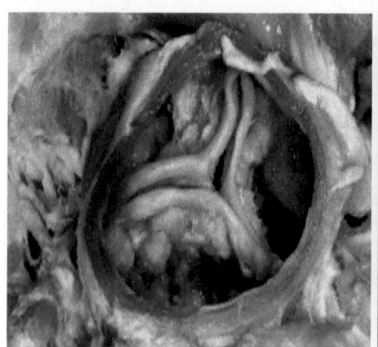 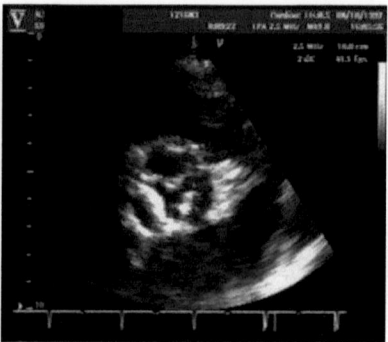

Figure 1: Tricuspid native aortic valve stenosis (Google).

Figure 2: Transesophageal echocardiogram showing a tricuspid, thickened, and severely stenotic aortic valve (AVA = 0.9 cm²) (Osrane k, et al, 2008).

Bicuspid aortic valve (BAV) is a congenital disorder associated with disturbed ascending aortic blood flow. Using a new strategy to dissect flow mediated gene expression, we identified several novel flows associated genes, particularly related to angiogenesis, wound healing and mechanosensing, showing differential expression in the ascending aorta between BAV and tricuspid aortic valve patients. Fifty five percent of the identified genes were confirmed to be flowresponsive in the rat aorta. A disturbed flow, and consequently an altered gene expression, may contribute to the increased aneurysm susceptibility associated with BAV morphology (Ohashi K L, et al., 2004).

Calcific deposits contribute significantly to the degree of stenosis in diseased aortic valves, and have been directly associated with a more rapid clinical progression of aortic stenosis. The widespread clinical application of echocardiographic imaging has made it possible to identify patients at earlier development stages of valve disease, raising the possibility for potential benefits associated with earlier valve treatment interventions (Ohashi K L, et al., 2004).

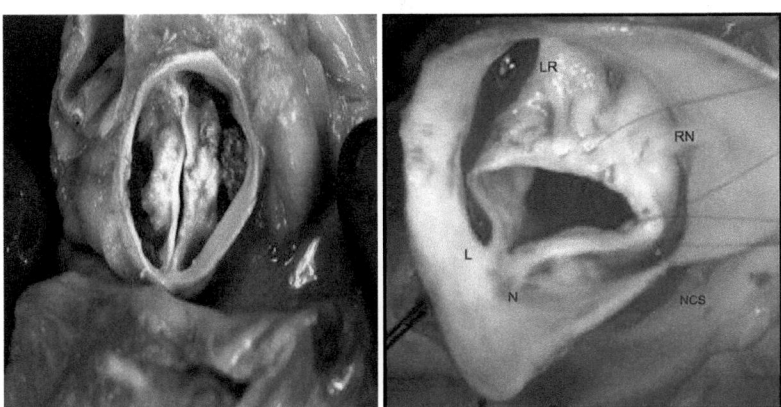

Figure 3: Native Bicuspid Aortic Valve (Google scholar). Figure 4: Native Unicuspid Aortic Valve (Google scholar).

Prosthetic Aortic Valves:

Aortic stenosis is the most common valvular disease requiring valve replacement with a prevalence of 2-4% in adults greater than or equal to 65 years of age. There is increasing evidence that AS is an active inflammatory process that is highly regulated, displaying multiple hallmarks of atherosclerosis. Clinically, the definite therapy of advanced AS is prosthetic valve replacement. Bioprosthetic tissue valves (BPs) possess superior thromboresistant and hemodynamic properties compared with mechanical valves. However, cusp degeneration and calcification also limit their long-term outcome. The pathogenesis of BP calcification as well as that of native valves is still poorly understood. Recent studies suggest a similar valvular pathology that underlies both types of valvular degeneration, but also an even more important role of inflammatory and repair processes in the case of BP degeneration. Prosthetic aortic valve includes, tissue prosthetic aortic valve and mechanical prosthetic aortic valve (see figure 5) (Skowasch D, et al., 2006).

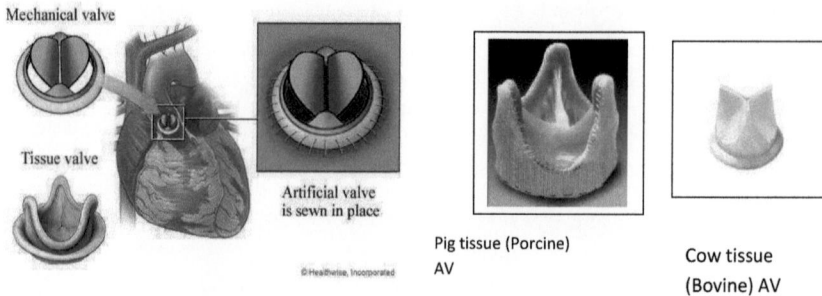

Pig tissue (Porcine) AV

Cow tissue (Bovine) AV

Figure 5: Picture of artificial (Tissue and Mechanical) AV sewn in places for AV replacement

Tissue Prosthetic Aortic Valve Stenosis:

The prosthetic aortic valve tissue can be obtained from the heart valve of pigs or the pericardium (sac surrounding the heart) of cattle (figure 5). The advantage of these types of valves is that it is normally only temporary or there would be no need for blood thinner. However, the disadvantage is that these valves may have a decreased structural durability compared to mechanical valves, causing earlier valve lifespan. In certain patients the valves may become calcified (restenosis) and stiff and malfunction in just a few years. The natural history of aortic stenosis can be affected by a number of comorbidities. Although renal failure is one of the known comorbidities for rapid progression of aortic stenosis, it is unclear whether hemodialysis alters the development and progression of prosthetic aortic valve stenosis (Mao M, et al., 2011).

Mechanical Aortic Valve Stenosis:

The mechanical replacement valve has the advantage that it lasts a long time without structural problems when compared to the tissue valves. However, the main disadvantages have to do with a need for lifelong blood thinner (anti coagulation drugs) to prevent blood clot formation on the valve. On the other hand, this will cause an increase in the chance of bleeding problems during the patient's lifetime, especially within elderly patients. Although most bleeding episodes are minor, there can be major bleeding complications which may require blood transfusions or may even be life-threatening. Without adequate thinning of the blood, there is an increased risk of blood clots forming on the valve, with the potential for these clots to break free into the blood stream. These free blood clots (known as emboli) may travel to distant organs in the body, such as travelling to the brain and a stroke may occur. Also, when emboli travel to an arm or leg, the limb could become cold, pulseless, motionless, and extremely painful and may travel to the heart and cause ischemic heart disease or myocardium infarction (MI) (Soyer R, et al., 1996).

Pathophysiology of Aortic Stenosis (AS)

Aortic stenosis is caused by restricted leaflet opening resulting from calcific changes of a normal trileaflet or congenitally bicuspid valve, or from rheumatic valve disease. Rheumatic valve disease is rare in the United States and Europe, although it is the most common cause of valve disease worldwide. Most cases of aortic stenosis are caused by a congenitally bicuspid valve that occurs in about 1% of all adults. Approximately 20% of patients with a bicuspid valve have significant regurgitation, requiring valve surgery at ages 20 to 40 years (figure 6) (Stout K K, et al., 2007).

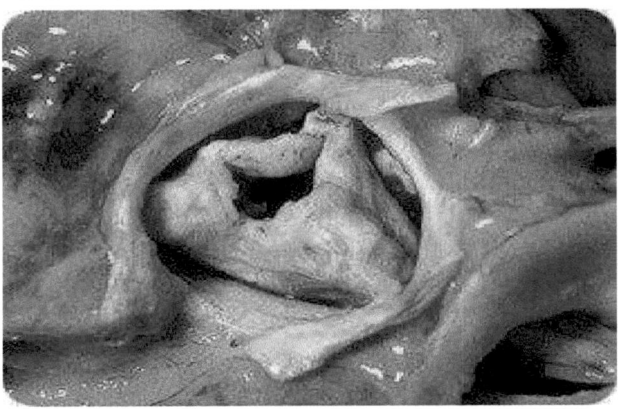

Figure 6: Native three cusped AS, resulting from Rheumatic Fever (Google scholar).

However, most have a relatively normal valve function until superimposed calcific changes result in deceased leaflet motion. A calcified bicuspid valve accounts for 60% of aortic valve replacement surgery in patients between 40 and 70 years of age and about 40% of valve replacements in patients over age 70 years. Progressive calcific changes resulting in stenosis of an anatomically normal trileaflet aortic valve usually do not require valve replacement until after age 70 years. The leaflet changes in calcific aortic stenosis are caused by an active disease process similar to atherosclerosis, characterized by lipid infiltration, inflammation, and tissue calcification. The presence of calcific valve disease is associated with clinical factors such as hypertension, male sex, smoking, hyperlipidaemia, and diabetes. In addition, genetic factors might play a role in disease initiation and progression. Although it has been proposed that treatment directed towards these clinical factors, such as lipid-lowering therapy, might slow disease progression, the single prospective randomized clinical trial reported to date did not find a significant effect of therapy on disease progression. Even if medical therapy might be beneficial early in the disease course, when severe stenosis is present, it is unlikely these changes can be reversed by medical therapy (Stout K K, et al., 2007).

The cause of an Aortic Stenosis Disease Aetiology:

The most common cause of AS in adults is calcification of a trileaflet or congenital bicuspid and unicuspid valve (see figure 1& 2). Calcific AS is a progressive pathology, starting with simple leaflet thickening, fibrosis then eventually severe calcification, small valve area and tight stenosis. The exact pathology of AS is not clearly understood. Studies have shown that the risk factors for AS are similar to those of atherosclerosis, hence the suggestion that the pathology is likely to be similar (Roberts WC, 1970; Lindroos M, et al., 1994; Stewart BF, et al., 1997).

Histological studies of valve specimens also demonstrated inflammation, lipid accumulation and fibrosis on the stenotic aortic valve, taking similar morphology to those seen in atherosclerotic disease. Less common causes of acquired AS are a rheumatic valve disease, although much less prevalent than rheumatic mitral valve disease (Somers, P, et al., 2006; Iung B, et al., 2007).

Rheumatic AS presents with typical pathological leaflets, thickened and calcified with fused commissures resulting in additional regurgitation. Isolated congenital AS is a rare pathology, with the bileaflet aortic valve being the commonest and sub or supra aortic valve stenosis the less common. Although it can result in similar pathophysiology, sub aortic membrane may cause severe narrowing of the left ventricular outflow tract (LVOT) early in life and cause a serious need for surgical removal. Finally, aortic valve stenosis should be differentiated from subarctic basal septal hypertrophy, causing LVOT narrowing and potential obstruction, particularly at a fast heart rate (Gersony WM, 2001; Henein. MY, et al., 1997).

There are many factors that may have a direct or indirect relationship with the acceleration or slow down the rate of aortic stenosis (AS) in both native (prosthetic valve) and artificial valve. Artificial tissue valve, from cows (Bovine) and from pigs (Porcine) or mechanical aortic valve. Ageing is one of the most common causes of deposits and buildup of calcium in the aortic valve in some older people, in 3% of people aged over 65 years, which is not clear yet why this happens. The other common cause is called Rheumatic Fever. It is a condition that sometimes occurs during a bacterium infection called the streptococcus (Busko M, 2011 European Society of Cardiology, European Heart Journal 2007; Osler W, 2000).

The studies have demonstrated that severe aortic stenosis occurs with an increased frequency in patients with renal failure. Abnormalities of the aortic valve are common in patients undergoing dialysis for chronic renal failure. Also, studies show that using computed tomography that calcification of the aortic valve is progressive in patients on dialysis. (Raine A, 1994; Maher. E, et al., 1987; Baglin A, et al., 1997; Perkovic V, et al., 2003).

Also, recent epidemiologic studies have revealed the risk factors associated for vascular atherosclerosis, including the male sex, smoking, hypertension, and elevated serum cholesterol, similar to the risk factors associated with the development of AV stenosis. An increasing number of models of experimental hypercholesterolemia demonstrate features of atherosclerosis in the AV, which are similar to the early stages of vascular atherosclerotic lesions. Experimental and clinical studies demonstrate that the hypercholesterolemic AV develops an atherosclerotic lesion which is proliferative and expresses high levels of osteoblast bone markers which mineralize over time to form bone. Calcification, the end-stage process of the disease, is necessary to understand as a prognostic indicator in the modification of this cellular process before it is too late (Rajamannan NM, 2010).

The other underlying causes of AS is, congenital valve abnormalities, such as unicusped or bicuspid which is caused by wear and tear of aortic valve (normal Aortic Valve is three cusps) (Busko.M, 2011 European Society of Cardiology European Heart Journal 2007; Osler W, 2000).

Sign and symptoms of AS:

Symptoms related to AS depend on the degree of stenosis. Most people with mild to moderate aortic stenosis do not have symptoms. Symptoms usually appear in those with severe AS. The most common symptoms of AS are; chest pain (angina) and chest tightness on exertion, feeling faint on exertion, shortness of breath (SOB) especially on exertion, felling fatigue, especially during times of increased activity and heart palpitations (felling of a rapid flattening heart beat or fibrillation and hearing a heart murmur) (Becher H, 2008).

Clinical Presentation of aortic stenosis:

Symptoms are the best indicator of the hemodynamic significance of stenosis in a given patient, as some patients might tolerate the same degree of stenosis very differently. Therefore, a careful history is crucial in deciding the appropriate course of therapy and the expected response to comorbid illnesses and medications. The classic symptoms of aortic stenosis are angina, syncope, and heart failure. Dyspnea usually is due to diastolic dysfunction caused by longstanding elevated afterload and increased filling pressures. Angina and, to a lesser extent, dyspnea are related to oxygen supply and demand mismatch caused by the hypertrophied ventricular muscle and

13

alterations in coronary blood flow without the pericardial coronary disease. Exertional syncope is presumed caused by inability to increase stroke volume in the face of increased demands of exercise. With fixed obstruction at the valve level being the primary component of ventricular afterload, the normal peripheral vasodilation with exercise results in hypotension and decreased cerebral perfusion, instead of the increase in stroke volume expected with a decrease in afterload (Stout K K, et al., 2007).

However, many patients will not report overt symptoms, but might instead simply notice a decrease in exercise tolerance without a discrete limiting symptom. This exercise intolerance can often be misinterpreted as "just due to aging" by patients and their providers but is in fact symptomatic aortic stenosis. Eliciting a history of symptomatic aortic stenosis requires asking specifically about exertional dyspnea, syncope, chest pain, and heart failure symptoms. Also necessary is a broad approach to assessing change in exercise tolerance over time (Stout. K K, et al., 2007).

Diagnosis of Aortic Stenosis (AS):
Physical Examination:

Aortic Stenosis (AS) is most often can be detected during routine examination of the heart and circulatory system.

Diagnostic Test Techniques:
Electrocardiogram (ECG):

ECG is the recording of electrical activity generated by the cells of the heart. Analysis of these recodes details allows diagnosis of a wide range of heart conditions. Broadening of the QRS complex duration, commonly seen in severe AS (Wanger S G, et al., 2008).

Chest X-ray:

Chest X-ray can assist in the diagnosis, showing calcific aortic valve and established diseases such as enlarged left ventricle and left atrium.

Cardiac Catheterisation:

It is the gold standard of diagnosing cardiovascular disease. Cardiac Catheterisation can provide a definitive diagnosis, indicating severe stenosis in valve area of (<0.8 cm2) (Rob. B, et al., 2007).

Echocardiography (Methodology and Techniques):

Echocardiography has emerged as a standard clinical tool in AS evaluation, quantification and serial examinations. 2D echocardiography allows evaluation of the LV chamber, ejection fraction (EF), wall adaptation and evaluation after load, visualisation of aortic valve leaflet and measurements Doppler quantification. Doppler echocardiography enables measurements of maximum aortic jet velocity, mean pressure aortic valve gradient and aortic valve area by continuity calculation. This measurements help to grate the AS severity into three grade severity, mild, moderate and severe. Aortic jet velocity is most reproducible measurement from these three Doppler echocardiography measures (See Figure below) (Jacob D P, et al 2008).

Echo is one of the best non-invasive tests to evaluate the heart anatomy and function. The study evaluated that for patients with very mild AS, it is very useful to follow with a non-invasive approach every 1 or 2 years, and an annual follow-up is suggested for patients with mild stenosis. Also, about one-third of patients with moderate stenosis at initial echocardiography examination appear to have severe stenosis after the following period. Therefore, they recommend that patients with moderate stenosis undergo non-invasive evaluation every 6 months. In addition, the study evaluates that aortic stenosis is more problematic than aortic replacement (AR) in children with congenital AVS even with probability of aortic restenosis. Doppler estimated mean gradient is very useful in predicting the need for intervention in children with AVS (Eroglu A G, et al., 2006).

The foundation idea in innovation of 3D-Echo was based on the principle that a 3D data set could be reconstructed from a series of 2D images. In this method a serial 2D images are obtained using either freehand scanning or a mechanically driven transducer. A series of images is obtained by manually tilting the transducer along a fixed plane, and a spatial locator attached to the transducer translates the 3D spatial location onto a cartesian coordinate system. The ability to extract hemodynamic information derived from 3D colour Doppler ultra sonography is currently being investigated (Hung J .MD et al., 2007).

CHAPTER TWO

LITRITURE

REVIEW

2.0 LITRITURE REVIEW:

Aortic stenosis (AS) will increase with the rise in an aging population and aortic valve replacements is the most common indication in adults with severe symptomatic of valvular obstruction which is the only effective treatment, nowadays. Calcific aortic stenosis has many characteristics in common with atherosclerosis, including hypercholesterolemia. Intensive lipid-lowering therapy does not halt the progression of calcific aortic stenosis or induce its regression (Joanna S, et al., 2005).

The study shows that, in asymptomatic patients with aortic stenosis, it appears to be relatively safe to delay surgery until symptoms increase, but, the outcomes may be different. The incidence of moderate or severe valvular calcification, together with a rapid increase in aortic-jet velocity, identifies patients with a very poor prognosis. These patients should be considered for early (AVR) rather than have surgery delayed until symptoms develop (Rosenhek R, et al., 2000).

The advantages of using Echocardiography technique are; non-invasive, easy to access anytime and any day, realized at the bedside of the patients, real time of result and interpretation, can be repeated as often as needed for monitoring, useful for diagnosing assessment and monitoring and follow-up patients (Otto C M, 2010).

The ability of echocardiography to provide early diagnosis and an accurate measurement of disease severity, has increased the knowledge in regard of the natural history of the AS disease process and allows to follow the individual patients over time, long before valve replacement is needed. The mild symptoms indicate AVR if severe obstruction is present. The study shows that the measurements of severity of AS is clinically important for three reasons. First, it shows the severity of obstruction to provide the data for decision making about timing of valve replacement. Second to provide the quantitative measure allows to prediction of AS progression. Third, which is most important, is to ensure the valve abstruction is cause of the patients symptoms (Otto C M, 2010).

2D and 3D-Echo Studies:

The study shows 3D- Echo has been applied for anatomic assessment of the aortic valve and root morphology and to calculate the valve area in aortic stenosis. The technique has been used to delineate aortic flow patterns and has demonstrated feasibility and accuracy in quantifying aortic regurgitation. Currently, the assessment of the severity of aortic valve stenosis is essential for an appropriate management of these patients with AS. One of the most important assessments is calculation of the LVOT area, which is normally estimated using 2D-echo from the diameter obtained from a long-axis view in the parasternal plane. 3D-Echo is a safe, non-invasive imaging modality that is complementary and supplementary to 2D imaging and can be used to assess cardiovascular function and anatomy in various clinical settings (Hung J MD et al., 2007).

Measurement of the LVOT area using 3D-echo is more reproducible than with 2D-echo. Therefore, probably 3D-Echo is more accurate method for the evaluation of LVOT area. 3D-echo techniques show that the LVOT has an elliptical form and that its circularity does not depend on size. It may be that 3D-echo can provide a more accurate classification of the degree of severity of aortic valve stenosis than 2D-echo technique (Leopoldo P I, et al., 2008; Hung J MD et al., 2007).

The most important and widely used method of Echo is for assessing the severity of aortic valve stenosis is calculation of the effective area using the continuity equation. However, the use of the 2D-echo method is not without its restrictions. The limitations of the technique itself may lead to obtaining inaccurate measurements. Recently, 3D-echo has been used, which has many advantages in the assessment of valve disease. For example, it allows measurements to be made of different cardiac structures in any special plane. (Leopoldo P I, et al., 2008).

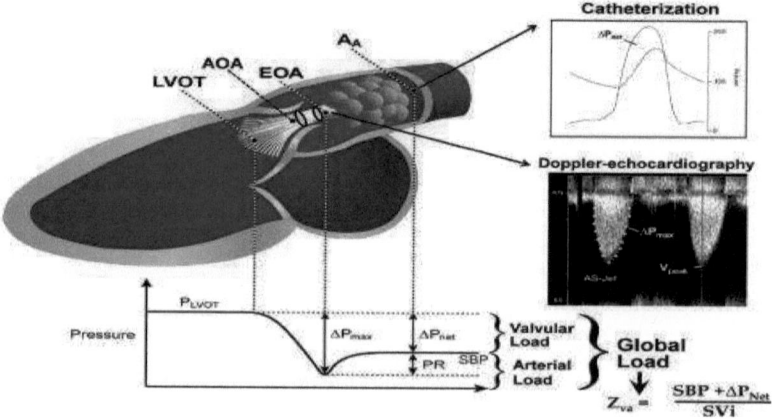

Figure 7: Blood flow from LV to Aorta through Aortic Valve (Pibarot P, et al, 2011).

Figure 7 shows, blood Flow and pressure across the left ventricular aortic tract (LVOT), though aortic valve, and ascending aorta during ventricular systole. When the blood flow contracts to pass through a stenotic orifice, the anatomic orifice area (AOA), a portion of the potential energy of the blood, namely, pressure, is converted into kinetic energy, namely, velocity, thus resulting in a pressure drop and acceleration of flow. Downstream of the vena contracta means the effective orifice area (EOA), a large part of the kinetic energy is irreversibly dissipated as heat because of flow turbulences. The remaining portion of the kinetic energy that is reconverted back to potential energy is called the "pressure recovery" (PR). In patients with medium or large size ascending aorta, the impedance can be calculated with the standard Doppler mean gradient in place of the net mean gradient. AA = cross-sectional area of the aorta at the level of the sinotubular junction; ΔPmax = maximum transvalvular pressure gradient recorded at the level of vena contracta (for example mean gradient measured by Doppler); ΔP net = net transvalvular pressure gradient recorded after pressure recovery (mean gradient measured by catheterization); LVOT = left ventricular outflow tract; PLVOT = pressure in the LVOT; SBP = systolic blood pressure; SVi = stroke volume index; V peak = peak aortic jet velocity; Zva = valvuloarterial impedance (Pibarot P, et al., 2011).

Figure 8, shows, superiority of LV Longitudinal Shortening over LVEF to Identify Myocardial Systolic Dysfunction in AS. The panels show the left ventricles (LV) of (A) a normal healthy subject, (B) a patient with aortic stenosis (AS) and normal myocardial function, and (C) a patient with advanced AS and myocardial dysfunction. The LV ejection fraction (LVEF) markedly underestimates the extent of myocardial systolic impairment in presence of LV concentric hypertrophy such as is often the case in AS patients (C). The increase in wall thickness associated with LV concentric hypertrophy results in a greater contribution of wall thickening to endocardia inward displacement (B and C). As a consequence, LVEF as well as any parameter based on endocardia displacement remains normal in presence of concentric hypertrophy, despite a significant impairment of intrinsic myocardial shortening and function (C). The longitudinal strain (LS) is thus more sensitive than LVEF to identify intrinsic myocardial dysfunction (Pibarot P, et al., 2011).

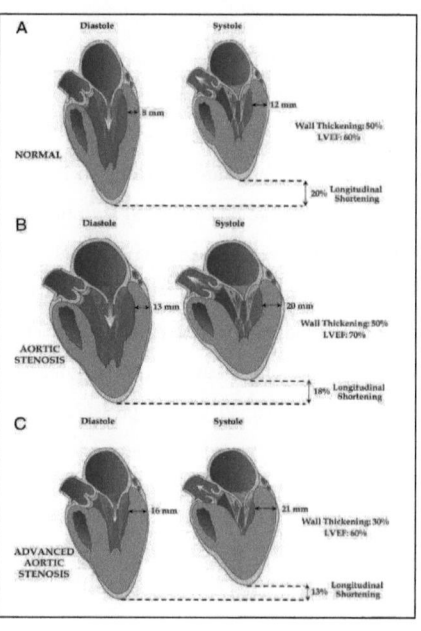

Figure 8: Left Ventricular Function LV/EF in normal and abnormal heart (Pibarot P, et al., 2011).

Causes and effects of Aortic Stenosis Disease (AS) (Pathology):

The aortic valve stenotic lesion implies an obstruction of forward blood flow through the valve and is caused by an abnormal increase in thickness and stiffness of the valve leaflet due to increased amounts of fibrosis and/or calcification, alternatively congenital or acquired fusion of the leaflets, resulting in a decreased effective valve orifice and in consequence, enhanced pressure load on the heart cavity and an increased blood flow velocity across the valve. In the case of the aortic valve one makes a distinction between aortic valve stenosis (AS) and aortic valve sclerosis. The latter implies a mild leaflet thickening without valve obstruction. Aortic valve sclerosis can be diagnosed by echocardiography as focal areas of increased echogenicity on the valve leaflets with normal valve motion and a normal, or only mildly increased integrate velocity across the valve. However, aortic valve sclerosis pressure, besides being a possible early stage of AS, comprises an increased risk of morbidity and mortality. The degree of aortic valve obstruction is generally classified arbitrarily into aortic valve sclerosis, for example; (mild leaflet thickening without valve obstruction), mild, moderate or severe stenosis. The regurgitate lesions are due to an inability of the valve to stay impenetrable when the pressure in front of the valve exceeds the pressure behind the valve (Rajamannan NM, et al., 2008).

In such regurgitate cases, the unidirectional flow cannot be maintained, instead the blood flows against the stream and thus increases the amount of blood the respective heart chamber has to cope with to maintain unchanged forward flow. Valve regurgitation can, in general, be caused either by a dilatation of the supporting valve ring making valve leaflet co-optation impossible, or by damages to the valve leaflets or their supporting structures. The degree of valve regurgitation is generally classified arbitrarily into the trace, (meaning barely discernable), mild, moderate or severe. As a result of the stenotic aortic valve, the left ventricle (LV) faces a significant pressure afterload which is known to affect LV structure and function as is the case with long standing hypertension. The raised intracavitary pressure raises, wall stress, which affects first the function of the subendocardial layer of the myocardium followed by the transmural layer. As the pressure increases and becomes significant, LV wall thickness increases and consequently the overall LV mass increases too. This is a potential compensatory mechanism to the LVOT obstruction and resistance as well as the exponential increase in wall stress, in order to maintain overall systolic LV functions (Krayenbuehl HP et al., 1988; Hess OM, et al., 1993; Takeda S, et al., 2001).

Since the disease is progressive, eventually subendocardial dysfunction occurs. The degree of subendocardial dysfunction usually correlates with the severity of the AS. This can easily be studied by accurate assessment of LV long axis function which reflects the subendocardium. Long standing conditions may result in irreversible subendocardial dysfunction, which affects the conduction system and hence broadening of the QRS duration, commonly seen in severe AS. The LV hypertrophy should then be seen as having a compensatory beneficial effect as well as a damaging effect on the subendocardium as it compromises its blood supply, hence a perpetual subendocardial ischemia even in the absence of epicardial coronary artery disease (Kupari M, et al., 2005; Takeda S, et al., 2001; Greenbaum RA, et al., 1981).

Left Ventricular hypertrophy and increase in muscle mass affects also diastolic cavity function and causes global slow relaxation. This is bound to affect the overall LV performance with most filling volume occurring during late diastole rather than early diastole as is the case in normal hearts. These functional disturbances have been shown by various echocardiographic techniques including M-mode and tissue Doppler. With further deterioration of diastolic LV function, the cavity becomes stiff and filling pressures rise, which affect further the subendocardial function and patients may develop rather serious arrhythmia as a result (Zaca V, et al., 2010).

Furthermore, raised LV filling pressures themselves destabilize the left atrial (LA) function and increase LA size, hence the potential development of atrial fibrillation (AF). Most patients with raised LA pressures present with exertional breathlessness and signs of secondary raised systolic pulmonary artery pressure. Finally, late ventricular disease results in a fall in LV systolic function as shown by reducing ejection fraction (EF) and development of heart failure symptoms and signs. These patients may present with masked signs of AS which, again, could be inappropriately diagnosed and managed. It should be mentioned that fast developing AS resulting from the aggressive leaflet calcification process usually causes disproportionate hypertrophy and fast pressure buildup in the LA and atrial arrhythmia will occur (Eichhorn P, et al., 1992).

Treatment and Managements of Aortic Stenosis:

The Management of asymptomatic patients with AS, remains a source of discussion. According to the American Heart Association (AHA) and European Society of Cardiology (ESC) guidelines, when the patient develops the symptoms such as dyspnoea on exertion, chest pain or syncope is indicated for aortic valve replacement (AVR). The presence of symptoms of severe AS is (class I) indication for AVR. However, an exercise tolerance test (ETT) provides contraindication in patients with severe AS and some other patients who are free of cardiac disease symptom. As a result of other extra-cardiac conditions such as lung disease, renal failure and diabetes this will increase the risk of morbidity and mortality (Ennezat P V, et al., 2009).

While mild and moderate AS are monitored and followed up by regular echocardiographic assessment, at the same time, severe AS is an indication for valve surgery particularly in symptomatic patients, according to the current guidelines. Asymptomatic patients with severe AS remain a dilemma, although evidence exists confirming a significantly poor clinical outcome, if left ventricle unattended to function. Another dilemma is symptomatic patients with only moderate AS, in the presence of good LV function. The general belief is that the native valve should be preserved for as long as possible. Such patients with moderate AS who are limited by symptoms, particularly those with additional systemic hypertension have been shown to have worse LV and LA function compared to those without hypertension (Garcia D, et al., 2007, Bonow RO, et al., 2008; Vahanian A, et al., 2007; Rahimtoola SH, 2008).

Controversies remain regarding the best management plan for such patients since most hypertension medications are vasodilators with their known effect on AS physiology. These patients with moderate AS are commonly seen in cardiology clinics and more critical studies need to be properly designed to determine best management policies for them. Treatment is generally not necessary in asymptomatic patients. In most patients, watchful is recommended in asymptomatic AS including those with severe disease. In moderate cases, echocardiography is performed every 1–2 years to monitor the AS progression, possibly complemented with a cardiac stress test. In severe cases, echocardiography is performed every 3–6 months. In both moderate and mild cases, the patient should immediately make a revisit or be admitted for inpatient care if any new related symptoms arise (Eroglu A G , et al., 2006).

Medication Treatments:

During treatment, patients suffer from AS, medication may only be used to help relieve symptoms of heart failure when the heart failure is developing. In general, any medical therapy has relatively poor effects in treating aortic stenosis (Chockalingam A, et al., 2004). **These include;**

Angiotensin-Converting-Enzyme Inhibitor (ACE-inhibitors): For aortic stenosis, ACE inhibitors and statins are the two controversial medications which have been tested. Limited evidence suggests that ACE-inhibitors might improve exercise tolerance in AS patients with preserved LV systolic function. However, ACE-inhibitors are known for their vasodilatory effect and hence are traditionally a contraindication because they reduce the peripheral resistance resulting in increased transaortic valve gradient and reduced coronary perfusion (Chockalingam A, et al., 2004).

Statins: The use of statins in AS is based on the shared risk factors, found in AS and coronary atherosclerosis. These findings lead investigators to hypothesize that the two conditions are similar, and AS should benefit from statins and reduction of low density lipoprotein (LDL) cholesterol as coronary atherosclerosis does. A number of observational studies and trials have been conducted to objectively test this hypothesis, but failed to prove it. The most important is the SEAS trial being the largest study, which showed no effect on severity of AS despite a successful fall in LDL with simvastatin and ezetimibe. A recent meta-analysis also showed that AS does not respond to statins. If the early hypothesis proves true, the failure of response to statins could then be explained on the basis of commencing them in already late matured disease and calcified leaflets. In fact, these findings are not surprising since they mirror the results of using statins in calcific coronary artery disease shown by a number of randomized trials and a recent meta-analysis, which showed no structural benefit (Henein MY, et al., 2010; Rossebo AB, et al., 2008; Teo KK, et al., 2011).

Beta blockers: The pressure gradient and its drastic effect on LV function are very well known. A resting gradient of 60 mmHg in an asymptomatic patient is likely to double with increase in heart rate. Therefore, beta blockers have traditionally been used for heart rate control in AS patients. In asymptomatic AS patients, it may be useful since it can potentially reduce sudden death, ischemic events or artial fibrillation (AF), but are poorly tolerated by severe AS patients (Desai PA, et al., 2011).

Modified Risk Factors:

In most asymptomatic patients, the risk of surgery is greater than the risk of watchful waiting, so that management includes patient education, periodic echocardiography, and cardiac risk factor modification includes, reduce LDL and increase HDL, losing weight and stop smoking. Also, patients with mild and moderate AS are advised to avoid strenuous activities such intensive exercise (Desai PA, et al., 2011).

Surgical treatments:

Aortic Valve Replacement (AVR):

The only definite treatment for patients, who suffer with severe AS, is valve replacements. This will significantly improve the prognosis in patients with symptomatic severe aortic stenosis. The study shows, during the 3 years follow up, 52% of asymptomatic patients with severe AS had symptoms develop had AVR or died. Also, patients with severe AS, without symptoms and with symptoms, who had undergone AVR, had a survival advantage when compared with asymptomatic patients who had medical management alone. In adults, undergoing surgery for AS, calcific AS accounts for

51%, bicuspid aortic valve for 36% and rheumatic disease for 9%. The aetiology of aortic valve regurgitation (AR) is multifactorial and includes, on the one hand diseases involving the aortic root, e.g. Marfans syndrome, degenerative aortic dilatation and spondyloarthropathies, on the other hand diseases involving the aortic valve, e.g. Rheumatic disease, infective endocarditis and bicuspid aortic valve (Bonow R, et al., 2005; Dare AJ, et al., 1993).

AVR is the conventional treatment for severe symptomatic AS. It is performed either in isolation or concomitantly with coronary artery bypass grafting (CABG) surgery, which is known to take place in almost 50% of patients with AS. The overall mortality of isolated AVR is 3-5% in patients below 70 years and 5-15% in older adults. After successful AVR, the long-term survival rate becomes close to that expected at age matched controls, symptoms are less marked, and quality of life is largely improved. Some patients may be completely discharged from cardiology clinics to be followed up in the community (Vahanian A, et al., 2007).

Various valve substitutes have been developed over the years, varying from mechanical, bioprostheses, homografts and autografts, with the objective of inserting the ideal valve which causes the least possible resistance to the left ventricle. Clear differences, advantages and disadvantages between them exist. The life span of the mechanical valves is the longest, but it has a need for lifelong anticoagulation with its known potential problems, particularly in the elderly. Anticoagulants are also difficult to manage appropriately in patients living in rural areas in developing countries, with poor anticoagulation control. The life span of the biological prostheses is around 10-15 years. Getting old, the bioprostheses disintegrate and causes fast developing significant aortic stenosis/regurgitation, which may need lifesaving redo valve replacement (Hammermeister K, et al., 2000).

The main advantage of bioprostheses is the lack of the need for using anticoagulants. Aortic homografts are ideal in terms of hemodynamics of the LVOT. They result in a similar clinical outcome to bioprostheses without a need for anticoagulation. It must be mentioned that homografts are the ideal valve substitute for patients with recurrent or resistant aortic valve endocarditis, particularly when mechanical valves have previously been used. Despite that, aortic homografts are known for their potential problems, including calcification and availabilities. Homografts do calcify at a similar rate to bioprostheses, but no exact predictors for aortic calcification have been identified yet. In order to offer an optimal aortic homograft service, a well-organized homograft bank needs to be established. Aortic autograft (Ross procedure) is another potentially viable valve substitute. The procedure involves replacing the calcified aortic valve by the patient's own pulmonary valve and

25

inserting a homograft in the pulmonary position. This operation is ideal for younger patients because it allows the patient's own valve to grow. Autografts do not need anticoagulation, but need homograft banks as well as optimally experienced surgeons who are trained to undertake such procedure (Hammermeister K, et al., 2000).

Mechanical prostheses have better long-term survival than biological prostheses mainly because of the absence of primary valve failure while bleeding complications are more frequent. On the other hand, biological prostheses have better hemodynamics than mechanical prostheses. Despite that, biological prostheses have no difference in the rate of LV hypertrophy regression at long-term follow-up compared to mechanical prostheses (Villa E, et al, 2006, Hammermeister K, et al., 2000; Thomson HL, et al., 1998).

For biological prostheses, the stentless valve has a greater reduction in peak aortic velocity and a greater increase in indexed effective orifice area than the stented valve, despite similar reductions of LV mass at intermediate and long-term follow-up after AVR. Similar findings are reported in a meta-analysis, which showed that although LV mass index is significantly lower in a stentless group after 6 months of AVR, differences disappear after 12 months. Full aortic root replacement and reimplantation of the coronary arteries either with the stentless or the homograft valve produces near-normal transvalvular velocities and less than the stentless implanted in the subcoronary position. The Ross procedure, compared with homograft aortic root replacement, improves survival in adults, and is associated with improved freedom from reoperation and quality of life in long-term follow-up. The proportion of patients who survive after the Ross procedure is similar to that in the general population. The autografts have better hemodynamic outcome which does not change during follow-up compared with homografts which have a steady increase in transvalvular pressure up to 13 years after surgery (El-Hamamsy, et al., 2010; Perez de, et al., 2005; Cohen G, et al., 2010; Kunadian B, et al., 2007; Melina G, et al., 2002).

Aortic Valve Replacement (AVR) in high-risk patients:

In elderly AVR patients, the early mortality is approximately 4%-9%. Studies have shown that the 5, 10 and 15 years late postoperative survival (68%, 34% and 8%) is lower than the expected in an elderly population (70%, 42% and 20%). While, the overall postoperative survival in elderly patients at low risk, is similar to that of age- and sex-matched general population. Although AVR in the elderly can be performed with acceptable mortality and excellent long-term survival and functional recovery, the European Heart Survey on valvular heart disease demonstrates that 33% of patients over 75 years of age are not considered for surgical AVR because of age and LV systolic dysfunction or other co-mobidities, such as kidney impairment, chronic obstructive pulmonary disease and neurological dysfunction. Another survey in U.S. shows that half of symptomatic AS patients with quoted operative risks of 5-12% did not undergo AVR mainly because of other co-morbidities. In severe AS patients with poor LV function, AVR has significantly better outcome compared to those treated medically. Undoubtedly, such patients are likely to carry a significantly higher surgical risk (amounting for up to 10%) compared to those with maintaining LVEF, with an estimated in-hospital mortality of 8-9%. However, the gain benefit in terms of clinical outcome outweighs the surgical risk. In fact, guidelines support AVR in such patients (Vahanian A, et al., 2007; Ashikhmina EA et al., 2011; Iung B, et al., 2005; Bach DS, et al., 2007; Kolh P, et al., 2007; Tarantini G, et al., 2003).

Clinical results after AVR surgical operation:

After a successful AVR, symptoms become less noticeable, if do not disappear, and the quality of life greatly improves. The long-term survival after 5, 10 and 15 years is 94.6%, 84.7% and 74.9% respectively. Factors affecting short-term mortality and long-term survival after AVR include age (≥70 years), New York Heart Association NYHA functional class III and IV, aortic regurgitation, concomitant CABG and AF. Patients in a good NYHA functional class I and II before surgery usually have low operative mortality and excellent long-term survival, not different from the expected in the control population. Despite various scores currently used to assess surgical risk, optimally timed AVR remains a dilemma for some patients such as the elderly and those with LV systolic dysfunction (Kvidal P, et al., 2000).

Aortic Valve Bypass (AVB):

The calcified AS is the most common valve disease within elderly people in the 8th or 9th decade of their life who often show associated co-morbidities like reduced LV function, impaired renal function, pulmonary hypertension, diabetes mellitus, stroke and other diseases. For this reason, in many cases pre-operative morbidity and mortality are too high for surgical valve replacement. Up to 30 % of patients were rejected to do valve replacement operation due to primary end point, which is the rate of death from any cause, therefore they will undergo aortic valve bypass (Leon M B, et al., 2010).

Balloon Valvuloplasty (BV):

Both the experience and the literature show that balloon aortic valvuloplasty is followed by an immediate improvement in hemodynamic status by a decrease in valve gradient and an increase in valve area. However, the hemodynamic benefit is typically short-lived, with a very high restenosis rate. Balloon aortic valvuloplasty is not an alternative to aortic valve replacement, which remains the best treatment for calcified aortic stenosis; the benefits and long-term results of aortic valve replacement are well established, even in the elderly. BV is being used for infants and children, where a balloon is inflated to stretch the valve and allow greater flow, this is may be effective. However, in adults, generally it is ineffective, as the valve tends to return to a stenosis state (Rob. B, et al., 2007; Soyer R, et al., 1996).

Transthoracic Aortic Valve Implantation (TAVI):

The study shows the durability of both the safety and efficacy of TAVI, using the self-expanding Medtronic Core Valve prosthesis for the treatment of patients with severe AVS. It shows after during two years follow up after the implantation procedure of pre-independent risk future, there was no any structure valve deterioration or significant changes of hemodynamic status of the prostheses valve. Moreover, TAVI is a novel therapy, which may be used as an alternative to standard surgical aortic valve replacement in the future. TAVI is a less invasive treatment for high-risk patients with aortic stenosis. Therefore, TAVI has been suggested for patients with severe aortic stenosis and coexisting conditions who may not be a candidate for surgical replacement of the aortic valve (Bielefeld. L, MD, et al., 2011).

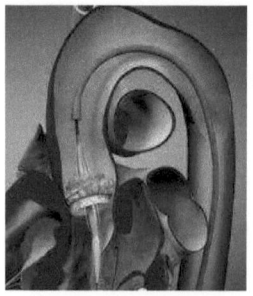 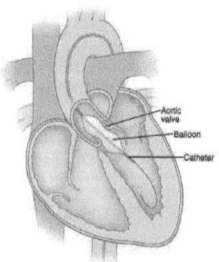 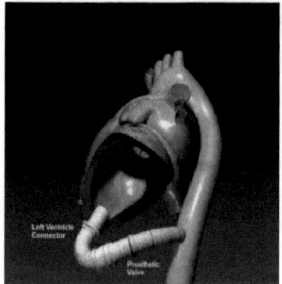

Figure 9: TAVI procedures (Google).

Figure 10: Aortic Balloon Valvoplplasty (Google).

Figure 11: Aortic Valve Bypass (Google).

Evaluation Disease Severity and Progression:

Aortic Valve stenosis severity is a continuum and not a single value defines clinically significant obstruction. Several other more sophisticated measures of aortic stenosis severity have been proposed, including stroke work loss, valve resistance, and valve impedance, but these measures are rarely used for clinical decision making. The result shows that, calcific aortic stenosis is a progressive disease. It appears that patients with aortic sclerosis progresses to significant stenosis in approximately 16% of adults within about 8 years. When even mild stenosis (defined as a Doppler aortic jet velocity 2.5 m/s) is present, the average rate of hemodynamic progression is an increase in jet velocity of 0.3 m/s per year, an increase in mean transaortic pressure gradient of 7 mm Hg per year, and a decrease in valve area of 0.1cm^2 per year (Stout K K, et al, 2007).

Consequence complication of Aortic Stenosis:

Aortic Stenosis may cause several consequence complications which may become severely life-threatening. This is including a Heart Failure, Chest Pain, Syncope, Irregular Heart Rhythm (arrhythmia), Endocarditic and Cardiac Arrest (Desmond. J. G et al., 2005).

CHAPTER

THREE

METHODOLOGY

3.0 METHODOLOGY:

3.1 Subjects:

A large-sized study sample will be used in this research trial. The sample size consists of 215 participants divided into three groups; the first group has 132 participants with native aortic valves, the second group has 46 participants with Tissue Prosthetic Aortic Valves and the third group has 37 participants with Mechanical Prosthetic Aortic Valves. All participants have been recruited from the NHS Hospital at Preston and Chorley Cardio-respiratory Departments, Lancashire Teaching Hospital Foundation NHS Trust, United Kingdom. Participants' in the trial will include both genders, and ages will vary from 21-92 years old.

3.2 AIMS:

The aim of this study is:

1-To evaluate, the result of diagnosis and the effect of the risk factors, on the progression of aortic stenosis, in native and artificial (mechanical & tissue) aortic valves, using the Echocardiography Technique.

2- To compare the progression of aortic valve stenosis, between native aortic valves and artificial (mechanical & tissue) aortic valves.

3.3 OBJECTIVES:

1- Carry out what risk factors may affect the rate progression of AS in the patients with native AV, using Echocardiography Technique.

2- Evaluate the rate of progression of AS in the patients with tissue prosthetic AV, using Echocardiography Technique.

3- Evaluate the rate of progression of AVS in patients with Mechanical Prosthetic AV using Echocardiography Technique.

4- Compare the rate of AS progression between the native AV, Tissue Prosthetic AV and Mechanical Prosthetic AV.

3.4 RESERCH DESIGN:

This research is a Non-experimental research design and does not involve a manipulation of the situation, circumstances or experience of the participants. Non-experimental research designs can be broadly classified into several categories, for this research, one of the categories, relational design by which a range of variables is measured, is being used. These designs are also called correlation studies, because correlation data are most often used in analysis. It is important to clarify here that correlation does not imply causation, and rather identifies dependence of one variable on another. Correlation designs are helpful in identifying the relation of one variable to another, and seeing the frequency of co-occurrence in two natural groups. Other, category of the research design being used in this research is comparative research. This design will compare two or more groups on one or more variables, such as the effect of age, sex, total cholesterol, HDL, TGL, LDL, max velocity, max gradient, mean gradient, cardiac rhythm, renal function and LV function on grades and progression of aortic stenosis.

3.5 PUPOLATION AND SAMPLES:

All subjects (215 patients) were recruited from the in patients and out patients at the Cardio-Respiratory Departement, Lanchashire Teaching NHS Trust (Preston). The patients are suffering from aortic valve stenosis. They are divided into three different groups of aortic valve patients (Native Aortic Valves, Tissue Prosthetic Aortic Valve and Mechanical Prosthetic Aortic Valves). The subjects selected are from the year 2000 until 2012. There were between 3 years and 11 years of measurement data available for each patient, depending on the severity and symptomatic progression and correlation of underlying causes.

3.5.1 INCLUSION CRITERIA:

The inclusion criteria are subjects (male and female) between 18 – 100 years. The patients are suffering from aortic valve disease and are under investigation/treatment at the NHS hospital. Each participant in the study must speak, read and write English to a standard level, and must read and sign a consent form (Spence S. 1989).

3.5.2 EXCLUSION CRITERIA:

The participants in the recruitment, assessment will be excluded from the trial if pregnant, or if they have pre-existing medical conditions or impairment which they consider may impair or impede their ability to participate in physical activity if needed (Dehghani M. et. al., 2004).

3.6 STUDY SETTINGS:

The study will take place within the Cardio-respiratory Department, Preston and Chorley Hospital (NHS Trust). At this site, there are 215 patients who suffer from aortic valve stenosis, native and artificial (mechanical & tissue) aortic valves, who are currently under investigation and treatment. The participant age was between 21-92 years old in both male and female. This information was obtained on behalf of a member of staff from the Cardio-respiratory Department at the hospital.

3.7 MATERIALD AND METHODS:

In the clinical trial, in order to ensure validity and reliability, the same quality of echocardiography and dimensional view (2-D) has been used. Also, in order to maintain the validity and reliability in the trial, participants will be fully informed about the nature of the trial and they will have to state that they understand the nature of the trial before signing the participant consent form (Silverman. D, 2004).

An echocardiogram can best determine the severity of the aortic valve disorder. If they are curious, the key determinants for classifying aortic stenosis are valve area, aortic velocity and mean pressure gradient. Therefore, Echocardiography is recommended to be used in the diagnosis and follow-up of AS patients and after intervention. The valve calcification is easily detected on the 2D imaging, but can only be qualitatively evaluated. Doppler flow velocity is conventionally used to evaluate the severity of valve stenosis, from which the peak transaortic valve velocity is measured. The aortic valve area (AVA) is then calculated from the LVOT diameter and velocity-time integral (VTI) using the continuity equation ($AVA=CSALVOT \times VTILOVT/VTIAV$). A simplified method is the direct comparison of the peak flow velocity in the sub-valve area and that across the aortic valve. Severe stenosis is present when the velocity ratio is 0.25 or less, corresponding to a valve area of 25% normal. This method has also been proved to be very accurate in confirming severe AS in patients with poor overall LV systolic function. The principles of imaging prosthetic valve function are similar to those used in the native valve (Baumgartner H, et al., 2009; Zoghbi WA, et al., 2009; Oh JK, et al., 1988).

Echocardiography and Positive Diagnosis of Aortic Stenosis (AS):

Aortic stenosis is suspected on two-dimensional images in patients with calcified and/or restricted aortic cusps. Valve calcifications appear as bright echocardiography images and show reflectivity of the aortic valve cusps (see figure 12) (O'Gara T, et at., 2006).

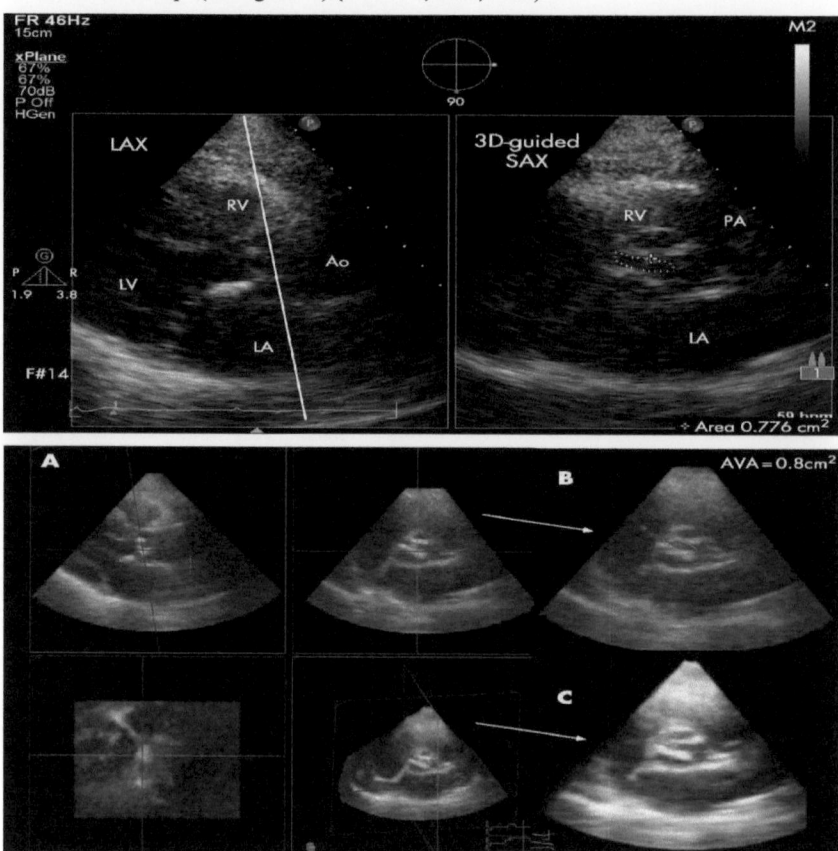

Figure 12: Parasternal long axis view, zoom on aortic valve, shows a severe calcifications of the aortic valve which almost does not open (AVA 0.8cm2) (O'Gara T . et at.. 2006).

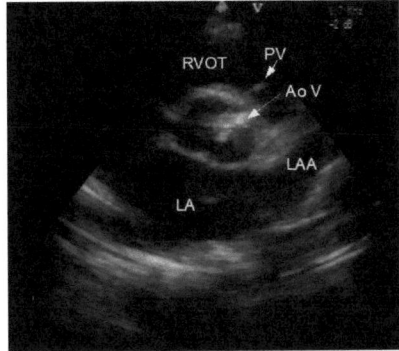

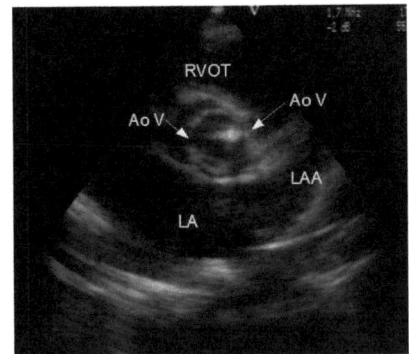

Figure 13: Aortic stenosis - parasternal short axis view - valve closed

Figure 14

Figure 14: Aortic stenosis in short axis view - valve open

in parasternal short axis view showing aortic stenosis with thickened aortic valve in closed position. RVOT: right ventricular outflow tract; Ao V: aortic valve; LAA: left atrial appendage; RVOT: right ventricular outflow tract; PV: pulmonary valve.

in parasternal short axis view. Valve is seen in open position with possible a single commissure which is thickened, suggestive of a unicuspid aortic valve. This picture was obtained after palliative balloon aortic valvotomy in a case with severe left ventricular failure, at high risk for open valvotomy / aortic valve replacement. Elective valve replacement is awaited. Pulmonary valve leaflet is not seen in this view as it is almost flush with the wall of the pulmonary artery in open position in systole.

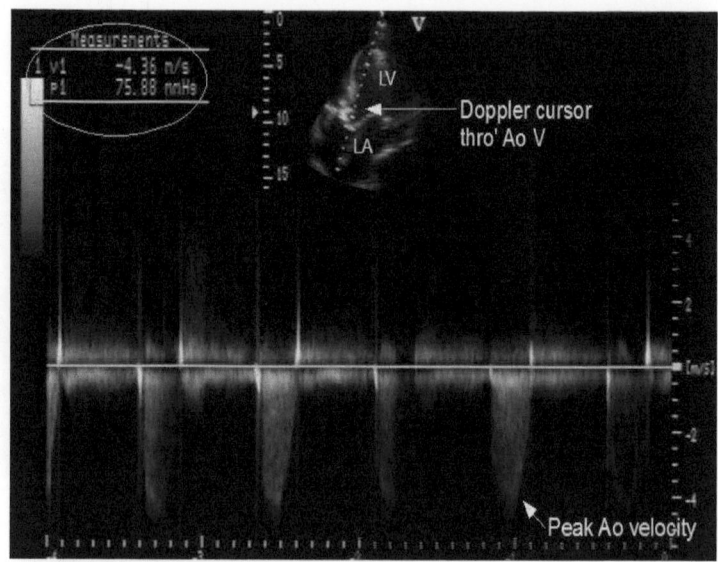

Figure 15: Continous wave (CW) Doppler imaging in aortic stenosis, show high peak aortic velocity (Francis J, 2008).

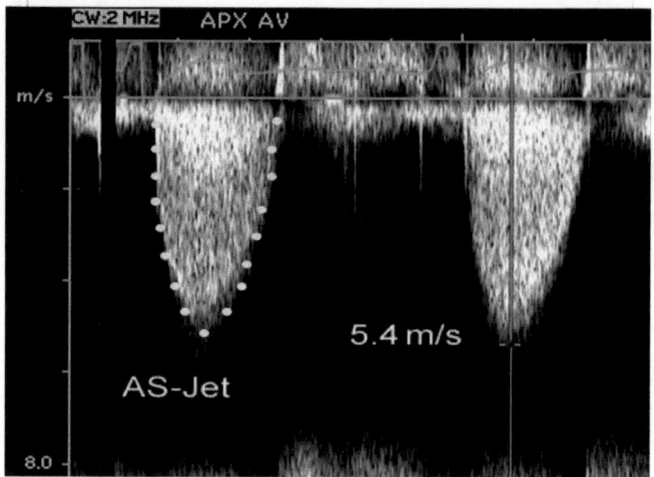

Figure 16: Continuous-wave Doppler of severe aortic stenosis jet showing measurement of maximum velocity and tracing of the velocity curve to calculate mean pressure gradient.

Maximum Velocity m/s of Aortic Stenosis jet velocity, CW Doppler (dedicated transducer):

Severe Aortic stenosis creates a high velocity jet of blood across the aortic valve as a result of the narrowing of the aortic valve area and left ventricular pressure. This high velocity jet can be imaged well only by continuous wave (CW) Doppler imaging as it will be well above the aliasing velocity for pulse Doppler. Aliasing velocity is the maximum velocity, which can be imaged by a given Doppler frequency and is dependent on the pulse repetition frequency. The highest velocity that can be detected is known as the Nyquist limit (figure 15 &16) (Francis J, 2008).

The CW Doppler cursor passes through the aortic valve in the apical five chamber view, on the side of (LA) left atrium and LV left ventricle (figure 15). The lower portion shows the tongue shaped Doppler signal due to systolic flow in the aorta just beyond the aortic valve at high velocity. The scale at the bottom represents a time axis and the vertical scale represents the velocity in m /sec. The scale beside the 2-D image at the top gives the depth in cm. Top left corner displays the measurements, in this case (figure 15) the peak aortic velocity (4.36 m/sec) and gradient (75.88 mm Hg), this is indicated severe aortic valve stenosis (Francis J, 2008).

Mean and maximum gradient data measurement:

Stenosis of the aortic valve creates an obstacle to aortic ejection; therefore a gradient of pressure between the left ventricle and the aorta will produce. This gradient of pressure can be measured, using Bernouilli law, by measurement of the maximum velocity across the aortic valve with continuous Doppler. In aortic stenosis, trans-aortic velocity is 3 to 5 m/s. To obtain the maximum gradient, use (caliper) it is an instrument used for measuring external or internal dimensions, to determine the maximum velocity of the regurgitant jet. The echocardiography machine will give the maximum gradient, derived from Bernouilli law. To obtain the mean gradient, use, trace to trace the envelope of the aortic outflow. The machine will calculate the area under the curve and will give you the mean gradient across the aortic valve (figure 17) (O'Gara T, et al., 2006).

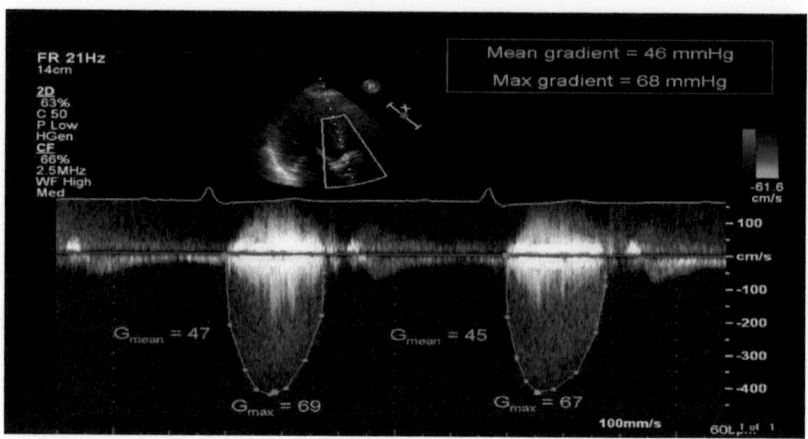

Figure 17: Severe aortic valve stenosis, Mean gradient=46mmHg, Max gradient=67 (ACC/AHA 2006 Guidelines)

Quantification of the degree of aortic stenosis is realized with continuous Doppler. To obtain an accurate measurement, it is crucial to optimize the alignment of the Doppler beam with the jet. The views which allow the best alignment are apical 5 and 3 chamber view. You can use colour Doppler to adjust the alignment of the Doppler beam with the maximum flow velocity (aliasing flow) (O'Gara T, et al., 2006).

The gradient is calculated from the velocity using the Bernoulli equation:

The mean gradient can be estimated by manually or electronically sketching out the envelope of the jet and the computer programme generates the mean gradient display. The gradient in this case is quite high, representing severe aortic stenosis. A limitation of assessing the severity by gradient alone is that the gradient may be falsely low when the left ventricle fails and is unable to generate adequate pressures. This can be seen in the Doppler tracing as a less steep slope of the tracing from the base to peak (Francis J, 2008; O'Gara T, et al., 2006).

Aortic Stenosis Category Measurements:

Aortic stenosis severity is best described by the specific numerical measures of maximum velocity, mean gradient, and valve area. However, general guidelines have been set forth by the American College of Cardiology Foundation (ACCF) and the American Heart Association (AHA) European Society of Cardiology (ESC). Writing committees are charged ACC/AHA and ESC for categorizing AS severity as mild, moderate, or severe to provide guidance for clinical decision-making. In most

38

patients, these three Level recommended parameters, in conjunction with clinical data, evaluation of aortic regurgitation (AR) and left ventricular (LV) functions are adequate for clinical decision-making. However, in selected patients, such as those with severe LV dysfunction, additional measurements may be helpful. Comparable values for indexing valve area and the dimensionless velocity ratio have been indicated in the (table 1 below), and the category of aortic sclerosis, as distinct from mild stenosis, has been added (Baumgartner H, et al., 2009).

Renal Function (normal and abnormal) Measurements:

The kidney has several functions, including the excretion of water, soluble waste, for examples, urea and creatinine and foreign materials, such as, drugs. It is responsible for the composition and volume of circulating fluids with respect to water and electrolyte balance and acid/base status. Measurements of renal function rely on measuring, in various ways the degree to which the kidney is successful in these roles mentioned above. The diagnosis of the underlying renal condition should be performed by a nephrologist. Also, general preventative measures require careful monitoring of renal function and protein excretion and are best undertaken under nephrology supervision. The earlier this prevention is performed, the greater the chance of avoiding the need for dialysis. In order to maximize the preventative potential, and to reduce the morbidity and mortality associated with chronic renal failure, the Evidence Based Practice Group (EBPG) feels that referral to the nephrologist should be made as soon as the glomerular filtration rate (GFR) drops to -60 mlumin. Estimation of the GFR is used clinically to assess the degree of kidney impairment and to follow the course of the disease, estimated GFR (ml/min/1.73 m^2). However, the GFR provides no information on the cause of the kidney disease. This is achieved by the urinalysis, measurement of urinary protein excretion, and, if necessary, radiologic studies and/or kidney biopsy. This requires the Nephrology departments to shift their focus from providing dialysis and transplantation in prevention and disease management (Stevens LA et al., 2006).

Cholesterol Measurements:

Cholesterol generally is known for being a bad thing, as high cholesterol is a major risk factor for heart disease, the leading cause of death in the United States, according to the Center for Disease Control. However, cholesterol is vitally important to hormone production and cellular health. There are several types of cholesterol includes LDL (Low Density Lipoproteins) flows through the blood stream carrying nutrients to the cell. LDL cholesterol is the so-called bad cholesterol because it deposits on the inside of your vessels to make plaques. Elevated levels of LDL increase your risk of heart disease and stroke. LDL cholesterol tends to stick to the walls of the blood vessels, leading to heart disease such as aortic stenosis, and other dangerous conditions. Another type of cholesterol called, High Density Lipoproteins (HDL), is considered the good lipid cholesterol, because when HDL flows through the bloodstream, it removes the LDL and prevents them from causing any problems (Birtcher K K, et al., 2004).

LDL and HDL Cholesterol Measurements

Low density Lipoprotein, LDL measurements is optimal below 100 mg/dl, (<2.6 mmol/L), with readings between 100 to 129 mg/dl (2.6-3.3 mmol/L) considered as above optimal, 130 to 159 mg/dl(3.3-4.1 mmol/L) considered as borderline, high will be ranged between 160 to 189 mg/dl (4.1-4.9 mmol/L) and above 190 mg/l (>4.9 mmol/L) considered as very high. Physicians recommend that men have HDL numbers no lower than 40 mg/dl (<1.03 mmol/L) for men and no lower than 50 mg/dl for women. The average man has an HDL level between 40 and 50 mg/dl, while the average woman has HDL levels between 50 and 60 mg/dl.

HDL cholesterol is the good cholesterol because a high HDL level decreases your risk of cardiovascular disease. For men, an HDL less than 40 is considered a risk factor for cardiovascular disease. For women, an HDL less than 50 is considered a risk factor for cardiovascular disease (Birtcher K K, et al., 2004).

Total Cholesterol Measurements:

Measuring total cholesterol requires a blood test that will then break down the total number of both LDL and HDL. The number is reported in milligrams per deciliter (mg/dl). Total cholesterol is the LDL and HDL readings combined. A total cholesterol reading below 200 mg/dl is optimal, and puts you at relatively low risk for heart disease. A reading of 200 to 239 mg/dl is considered borderline high risk; it is possible to have a reading in this range with normal levels of LDL balanced with high HDL numbers. Though the ratio is good, it is still recommended by the American Heart Association, that, patients have to work with the doctor to lower their total cholesterol under 200 mg/dl. Total cholesterol measurements above 240 mg/dl are considered high risk. People with total cholesterol readings above 240 mg/dl have more than twice the risk of coronary heart disease than people with readings below 200 mg/dl (Birtcher K K, et al., 2004).

Blood Plasma Triglyceride Measurements:

The detection of hyperlipidima depends upon blood sampling. Cholesterol estimates can be undertaken in a non-fasting state, but some other lipid measurements such as triglyceride require the fasting of the subject. A single measurement is not enough to make a decision, because accuracy of the method and because of variability in the cholesterol level from a time to time. Therefore if a high level of cholesterol is suspected, repeated measurements should be obtained especially if the patients drug lipid lowering includes HDL. The 6.0 mmol.L of cholesterol level, without the other risk factors, is associated with good prognosis, while a much lower value is associated with high risk of disease in patients with other risk factors like smoking and high blood pressure. Triglycerides are chemical compounds digested by the body to provide it with the energy for metabolism. Triglycerides are the most common form of fat that we digest, and are the main ingredient in vegetable oils and animal fats (Julian D G, et al., 2005).

How is triglyceride levels measured?

Triglyceride levels in the blood are measured by a simple blood test. Often, triglycerides are measured as part of a lipoprotein panel (lipid panel) in which triglycerides, cholesterol, HDL and LDL are measured at the same time. Patients have to be fasting for 9-12 hours before the test is required. Fat levels in the blood are affected by recent eating and digestion. Falsely elevated results may occur if the blood test is done just after eating (Julian D G, et al., 2005).

What are normal triglyceride levels, and what does high triglyceride levels mean?

Elevated triglycerides place an individual at risk for atherosclerosis. Triglyceride and cholesterol levels are measured in the blood to provide a method of screening for this risk. People who are very overweight, eat a lot of fatty and sugary foods, or drink too much alcohol are more likely to have a high triglyceride level. People with high triglyceride levels have a greater risk of developing cardiovascular disease including Aortic Valve stenosis. The normal triglyceride levels in the blood are less than 150 mg per deciliter (mg/dL). The borderline levels are between 150-200 mg/dL. The high levels of triglycerides (greater than 200 mg/dl) are associated with an increased risk of atherosclerosis and therefore coronary artery disease and stroke. The extremely high triglyceride levels (greater than 500mg/dl) may cause pancreatis disease (inflammation of the pancreas) (Julian D G, et al., 2005).

Severity	Jet velocity (m/s)	Maximum Gradient mmHg	Mean Gradient mmHg	LV/EF	Renal Function ml/min/1.73 m²	Total Cholesterol mg/dl	LDL Mm ol/l	HDL Mmol/l	TGL	Rhythm	AVA
Normal	<2.0	< 29	<17	58-70	>90	<200	<2.6		<150	NSR	3-5cm²
Mild	2.0-2.9	30-39	17-25	50-55%	60-89	200-240	2.6-3.3	<1.03	150-200 mg/dl	AF	2.5-1.5 cm²
Moderate	3.0-3.9	40-63	25-40	30-50%	44-59	240-280	3.3-4.1	1.03-1.55	>200 mg/dl	AF	1.5-1.0 cm²
Severe	≥4	≥ 64	>40	<30%	15-29	>280	4.1-4.9	>1.55	>500 mg/dl	AF	<1.0 cm²

Table 1: Assessments of Severity Aortic Valve Stenosis.

Left Ventricular Function and Ejection Fraction LVF/EF Measurements:

The other haemodynamic measurements of severity such as valve resistance, LV percentage stroke-work loss, and the energy-loss coefficient are based on different mathematical derivations of the relationship between flow and the transvalvular pressure drop. The effects of coexisting conditions, an assessment of severity. When LV systolic dysfunction co-exists with severe AS, the AS velocity and gradient may be low, despite a small valve area, a condition termed 'low-flow, low-gradient AS' as a result of less left ventricular hypertrophy (LVH) or cardiomyopathy (Baumgartner H, et al., 2009).

The most commonly used measure of cardiac function is the left ventricular ejection fraction (EF) assessment. This is can be performed with proportion of blood pumped out of the left ventricular during each cardiac cycle. Therefore, to calculate EF, the volume of the left ventricle at the end of diastole and systole, have been to estimated (Becher H, 2008).

Patients with poor LV systolic function may present with a low-flow, low-gradient state (effective aortic valve are will reduced to less than 1cm (AVA <1.0cm²) and reduce left ventricular function and ejection fraction, (LVEF <40%) and mean gradient pressure <30-40mmHg), peak gradient across the valve becomes not accurately representative of the stenosis severity. Mild-to-moderately diseased valves may not open fully due to depressed LV function, resulting in a functionally small valve area which is indicating pseudo severe AS. Therefore, patients may suffer from severe aortic valve stenosis despite of low aortic jet velocity and low maximum gradient and mean gradient grades as the result of left ventricular impairment. In these patients dobutamine stress echocardiography is recommended to differentiate true severe AS from pseudo severe AS (Vahanian A, et al., 2007).

Calculation of LVEF has important diagnostic, prognostic, and therapeutic implications, and a rapid, accurate, reproducible, and noninvasive method of calculating it would be desirable. Tow Dimensional echocardiography (2D Echo) is a widespread technique for clinical evaluation of LVEF. However, assessment of LV performance of 2-D echocardiographic techniques is based on geometric assumptions. Accurate measurement of LV volume and function requires the reconstruction of the true geometry of the heart, particularly in patients with distorted LV geometry and impaired LV function (Nosir F M, et al., 1996).

Echocardiographic studies were performed with a transducer system in the apical position while the patient lay comfortably in the 45° left recumbent position. To acquire cross-sectional images for reconstruction, the operator must find the centre axis around which the imaging plane is rotated to encompass the entire LV cavity. The movement of the transducer must be avoided, because the spatial coordinate system changes with transducer movement. Inadvertent patient movement during image acquisition can be prevented, for the most part, by thoroughly explaining the procedure to the patient before the test started. The examination, including the calibration procedures, selection of the optimal gain settings and conical volume with a few test runs, and the actual image acquisition, requires approximately 8 to 10 minutes in patients with sinus rhythm (Nosir F M, et al., 1996).

The Ejection Fraction (EF) is the volume of blood within a ventricle immediately before a contraction is known as the end-diastolic volume (EDV). Similarly, the volume of blood left in a ventricle at the end of contraction is end-systolic volume. The difference between end-diastolic volume (EDV) and end-systolic volumes (ESV) is the stroke volume, the volume of blood ejected with each beat. Ejection fraction (EF) is the fraction of the end-diastolic volume that is ejected with each beat; that is, it is stroke volume (SV) divided by end-diastolic volume (EDV):

EF=SV/EDV× 100=EDV-ESV/EDV
SV=EDV-ESV

The ejection fraction is commonly measured by echocardiography, in which the volumes of the heart's chambers are measured during the cardiac cycle. Ejection fraction can then be obtained by dividing stroke volume by end-diastolic volume as described above (Nosir F M, et al., 1996).

Accurate volumetric measurement of performance, of the right and left ventricles of the heart, is inexpensively and routinely echocardiographically interpreted worldwide as a ratio of dimension between the ventricles in systole and diastole. For example, a ventricle in greatest dimension could measure 6cm while in least dimension 4cm. Measured and easily reproduced beat to beat for ten or more cycles, this ratio may represent a physiologically normal EF of 60%. The normal range of EF is between 55-70% (Nosir F M, et al., 1996).

Dobutamine stresses, provides information on the changes in aortic velocity, mean gradient, and valve area, as flow rate increases, and also provides a measure of the contractile response to dobutamine, measured by the change in SV or EF. This data may be helpful to differentiate two clinical situations. First, is severe AS caused LV systolic dysfunction. Second, because the transaortic velocity is flow dependent; so the LV failure can lead to a patient with severe AS having an apparently moderate transaortic peak velocity and mean pressure gradient associated with a small effective orifice area. In this situation, aortic valve replacement will relieve afterload and may allow the LV ejection fraction to increase towards normal value (Baumgartner H, et al., 2009). Second, is a Moderate AS with another cause of LV dysfunction (e.g. Myocardial infarct or a primary cardiomyopathy). The effective orifice area is then low because the LV does not generate sufficient energy to overcome the inertia required to open the aortic valve to its maximum possible extent. In this situation, aortic valve replacement may not lead to a significant improvement in LV systolic function. A patient with a low ejection fraction but a resting AS velocity 4.0 m/s or mean gradient 40 mmHg does not have a poor left ventricle (LV). When the ventricle is demonstrating a normal response to high afterload (severe AS), and ventricular function will improve after relief of stenosis, the patients do not need a stress echocardiogram (Baumgartner H, et al., 2009).

3.8 PROCEDURES:

The data measurements are collected from 330 patients within three different groups of aortic valve patients (Native Aortic Valves, Tissue Prosthetic Aortic Valve and Mechanical Prosthetic Aortic Valves). Only 215 patients have chosen from all three groups, which are more suitable for medical statistical analyses. The subjects selected are from 2000 - 2012, who are suffering from Aortic Valve Stinosis. There is between 3 years and 11 years of measurements data available from each patient, depending of the severity and symptomatic progression and correlation of underlying causes.

The participants have been recruited from the Cardio-respiratory Department, Preston or Chorley Hospital (NHS trust). To follow Hospital guidelines, the participants will be approached through consent forms and will be informed about the investigation, their involvement, and its duration. A step-by-step approach will be incorporated into the test. The measurement will be recorded before and after performing all tests within each subject, then the results will be compared within the subjects and between subject groups. The subjects are all from in patients and out patients from Cardio- Respiratory Departments, Lancashire Teaching NHS Trust Hospital, which are suffering from aortic valves stenosis.

There were 15 different data measurements collected from all three groups of patients which are correlated with the rate progression and symptoms of Aortic Valve Stenosis, tese includes; Total Cholesterol Level, High density lipoprotein HDL, low density lipoprotein LDL, triglyceride TGL, Left Ventricular Ejection Fraction LVEF, aortic valve area (AVA), age, sex, Max Violcity M/S, Maximum Gradinat mmHg, Mean Gradient mmHg, Cardiac Rhythm, Patients groups, category of aortic valve stenosis (severity) and renal function.

3.9 DATA ANALYSIS:

As a result of the prediction of Disease Group Classification Status from Maximum Velocity, Maximum Gradient, Mean Gradient, LVF/EF, Age, and Total Cholesterol, HDL-Cholesterol, LDL-Cholesterol and Triacylglycerol Levels as Quantitative Explanatory, Active Variables, and Gender, Rhythm Status, Renal Function Status, and Category as Qualitative Explanatory Variables using Discriminatory Analysis (DA) used within analysis this research.

Quantitative Explanatory research can be defined as a method or style of research in which the principal objective is to know and understand the trait and mechanisms of the relationship and association between the independent and dependent variable. Discriminant function analysis is a statistical analysis to predict a categorical dependent variable (called a grouping variable) by one or more continuous or binary independent variables (called predictor variables). Discriminant analysis is a statistical procedure which allows us to classify cases into separate categories to which they belong on the basis of a set of characteristic independent variables called predictors or discriminant variables. The target variable (the one determining allocation into groups) is a qualitative (nominal or ordinal) one, while the characteristics are measured by quantitative variables. DA looks at the discrimination between two groups. Multiple discriminant analysis (MDA). MDA is a statistical technique used to reduce the differences between variables in order to classify them into a set number of broad groups and allows for classification into three or more groups (Sun J et al., 2012).

3.10 ETHICAL CONSEDERATION:

Any proposal involving research with human participants needs to consider the ethical aspects of the proposed study, and therefore an informed consent form and a precipitant consent template form will be issued to the relevant Ethics Committees for approval. Since the participants will be recruited from Chorley and Preston Hospital, the trial will require the approval by the Head of the Cardio-respiratory Department Ethics Policy Group. Therefore, there must be a request for ethical approval, through submission of an application form at the Cardio-Respiratory Department called (Lancashire Teaching Hospital NHS Foundation Trust Audit Registration Form). A copy of the form is shown below:

LANCHASHIRE TEACHING HOSPITAL NHS FOUNDATION TRUST
AUDIT REGISTRATION FORM

Directorate: Medicine

Audit title: The Diagnosis of Aortic Stenosis in Native and Artificial Aortic Valves using Echocardiography Technique.

Participants:	Job title:	Email address:	Bleep/Ext
Gaffor Omer	Student	go1cmr@bolton.ac.uk	

Mentor:

Trust Mentor: Shahid Tagari.

University of Bolton Mentor: Professor. Martin Grootveld

Directorate Audit Lead Signature: Susan Baxter

Audit rationale: (Why are you doing this audit?)

The aim of this study is to evaluate the result of diagnosing aortic stenosis in native and artificial aortic valves using Echocardiography ultrasound (with both 2D-Echo and 3D-Echo views).

Audit objectives: (What do you hope to achieve as a result of the audit?)

(1) To investigate the factors that may affect the rate of progression of Aortic Stenosis in patients with Aortic Stenosis using Echocardiography ultrasound with both 2-D and 3-D echo views.

(2) Analysis of the results of Aortic Stenosis progression in each subject and between the subjects using Echo technique.

(3) Investigation of any correlations between the results of using each of 2-Dimentional and 3-Dimentional Echocardiography view techniques.

(4) Evaluate the difference between the Aortic Valve Areas in patients with Aortic Stenosis and normal Aortic Valve.

Source of data collection: e.g. time frame & type of patients

Retrospective (please circle):

-The patients under investigations and managements of Aortic Valve Steniosis and   patients with normal Aortic Valve.

-Last five years of (Retrospective) data collection.

Details of any guidelines you will be auditing against:

British Cardiovascular Society (BCS) guideline.

	YES	NO
Assistance required from audit department		
Identification of patients		NO
Retrieval of casenotes		NO
Design of data collection pro-forma or questionnaire		NO
Data analysis		NO
Production of audit report or presentation		NO

Have patients been consulted in the planning or design of this audit?   NO

Date you hope to have audit completed by: September 2012

Date form completed: 07/02/2011

Table 2: LANCHASHIRE TEACHING HOSPITAL NHS FOUNDATION TRUST AUDIT REGISTRATION FORM

All participants will be provided with an outline of the information required for the purpose of the study, and will be asked to complete and sign an informed consent form. Patients will be advised that they can withdraw from the study at any time. All information will be kept strictly confidential and the participants will not be named, and data relating to them will be coded (Avci I. et. al., 2008).

Information will be held securely in password-accessible files. Informed consent will be obtained from all patients after the nature of the examinations are explained fully. The trial will not be harmful, and this will be explained to the willing and eligible participants. If a participant encounters a bad reaction during the investigation, he/she will be withdrawn from the study; medical care will also be covered includes: resuscitation and emergency life support (Fournier L. S. et. al., 2008).

Moreover, it is important to adhere to ethical norms in research because; firstly, ethical approval norms, promotes the aims of research, such as truth, knowledge and reduction or avoidance of error. Secondly, ethical standards, promote the values that are essential to collaborative work, such as trust, accountability, mutual respect and fairness. Because often research involves, a great deal of cooperation and coordination, among many different people, in different disciplines and institutions. Thirdly, many of the ethical norms help to ensure the researchers can be held accountable to the public. Fourthly, ethical norms of research also, help to build public support for research, because people are more likely to find a research project if they can trust the quality and integrity of research. Finally, many of the norms of research, promote a variety of other important moral and social values such as social responsibility, human rights, animal welfare, compliance with the law and health and safety (Fournier L. S. et. al., 2008).

CHAPTER FOUR

RESULTS AND

DISCUSSION

4.1 RESULTS:

Prediction of Disease Group Classification Status from Maximum Velocity, Maximum Grad., Mean Grad. LVF/EF, Age, and Total Cholesterol, HDL-Cholesterol, LDL-Cholesterol and Triacylglycerol Levels as Quantitative Explanatory, Active Variables, and Gender, Rhythm Status, Renal Function Status, and Category as Qualitative Explanatory Variables using Discriminatory Analysis (DA)

Data acquired were subjected to discriminatory analysis using maximum velocity, maximum grad, mean grad. LVF/EF, age, and total cholesterol, HDL-cholesterol, LDL-cholesterol and triacylglycerol levels as quantitative explanatory, active variables, and gender, rhythm status, renal function status, and category as qualitative explanatory variables (monitoring year was obviously excluded since this is a non-contributory variable). The two components (factors) derived from 3 treatment classifications (F1 and F2) displayed eigenvalues of 1.133 and 0.615 [Figure 18]. The first component accounted for 64.8% of the total variance, and when combined, components 1 and 2 accounted for 100% of the total variance. The variables included and their corresponding factor loadings (correlations) are given in Table 3 below. In interpreting the pattern, an item was considered to significantly load on a given component if the magnitude of the factor loading was ± 0.30 or greater for that component. Utilising this criterion, the active variables age, maximum velocity, maximum grad., mean grad, abnormal renal function and severe category were found to positively load on the first component, and normal renal function negatively loaded on it. Normal renal function and the mild category positively loaded, and maximum velocity, maximum grad., mean grad., abnormal renal function and severe category negatively loaded, on the second component. The significant contributions of some of the variables to both of the components are ascribable to the effects of the involvement of quadratic and/or first-order interaction variables in this model.

Determination of multicollinearity statistics demonstrated that there were only multicollinearity problems for the variables max. grad., mean grad., and toatl chlolesterol and LDL cholesterol levels only [VIF values ≥ 10; values of this parameter which are ≥ 10 indicate a significant level of multicollinearity].

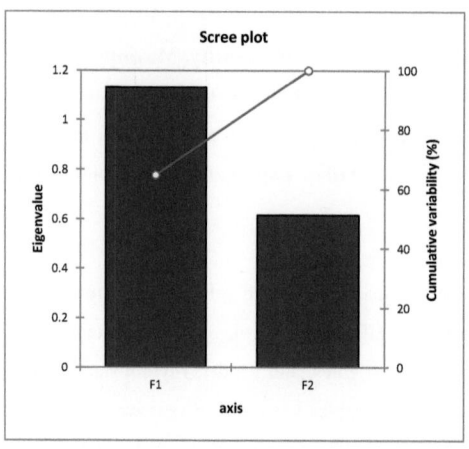

Figure 18: Scree89 Plot showing Eigenvalues as a function of the two factors derived from the model.

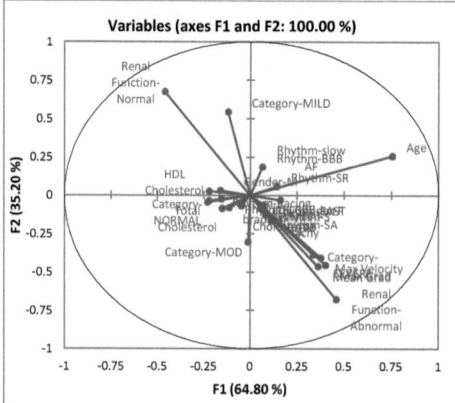

Figure 19: Canonical Correlation Analysis (CCA) plot showing inter-relationships between the variables incorporated into the experimental model (both qualitative and quantitative). This diagram shows that (1) the variable age is strongly correlated with Factor 1, (2) the MILD category and normal renal function variables are correlated with each other and Factor 2, and (3) the SEVERE category, abnormal renal function, and the mean and maximum grad. Parameters and the maximum velocity variable were all highly correlated with each other.

Table 3

Variables/Factors correlations:

	F1	F2
Age	0.755	0.258
Max Velocity	0.377	-.406
Max Grad	0.401	-.454
Mean Grad	0.362	-.463
Total Cholesterol	-.151	-.086
TGL	0.109	-.164
HDL Cholesterol	-.221	0.027
LDL Cholesterol	-.113	-.081
LVF/EF	0.070	-.065
Gender-M	-.161	0.031
Gender-F	0.161	-.031
Rhythm-AF	-.049	-.069
Rhythm-1st AVB	0.057	-.087
Rhythm-SR	0.142	0.058
Rhythm-SA	0.080	-.123
Rhythm-FAST AF	0.057	-.087
Rhythm-S tachy	0.080	-.123
Rhythm-slow AF	0.065	0.186
Rhythm-BBB	0.065	0.186
Rhythm-S brady	-.221	-.035
Rhythm-LBBB	-.156	-.025
Rhythm-Pacing R	-.221	-.035
Renal Function-Normal	-.459	0.676
Renal Function-Abnormal	0.459	-.676
Category-MOD	-.013	-.303
Category-NORMAL	-.230	-.045
Category-MILD	-.119	0.544
Category-SEVERE	0.336	-.385

As expected, the covariance matrices differed for at least two of the test groups investigated (Box tests performed with both χ^2 and Fisher's asymptotic approximations, Kullback's test, $p < 0.0001$ in each case), and hence the quadratic/interactive explanatory variable model was employed.

In total, 433 variables were isolated, although it should be noted that only two components (factors) were derivable therefrom since there were only three patient group classifications involved.

A canonical correlation plot revealed the nature of correlations between each of the explanatory variables incorporated into the model and the two factors [F1 and F2, Figure 18].

Of particular interest to this investigation is the significance of each contributory (explanatory) variable towards the clear discrimination between the three disease classifications evaluated. Firstly, a series of statistical tests were performed in order to determine differences between the means vectors of the three disease classifications, specifically the computation of Mahalanobis, Generalised Squared and Fisher distances, the Wilks-Lambda test (with Rao's approximation), Pillai's and Hotelling-Lawley's traces, together with Roy's greatest root. Results acquired demonstrated extremely highly significant differences between the means vectors of each disease group. Secondly, unidimensional tests of the equalities of Disease Class mean values were conducted, and it was found that the explanatory variables age, max. velocity, max. grad., mean grad., renal function and the mild and severe categories were all extremely highly significant 'between-Disease Groups' ($p < 0.0001$), and HDL cholesterol, moderate category and S brady and Pacing R rhythm varaiables were also highly significantly different ($p = 0.024$, 0.007, 0.023 and 0.023 respectively) (Table 4). Therefore, it was concluded that all these variables very highly significantly contributed towards the discrimination between the three classifications investigated in the clinical trial.

Table 4 Unidimensional test of equality of the means of the classes:

Variable	Lambda	F	DF1	DF2	p-value
Age	0.672	68.555	2	281	< 0.0001
Max Velocity	0.862	22.540	2	281	< 0.0001
Max Grad	0.836	27.540	2	281	< 0.0001
Mean Grad	0.849	25.059	2	281	< 0.0001
Total Cholesterol	0.985	2.134	2	281	0.120
TGL	0.983	2.360	2	281	0.096
HDL Cholesterol	0.974	3.785	2	281	0.024
LDL Cholesterol	0.991	1.323	2	281	0.268
LVF/EF	0.996	0.594	2	281	0.553
Gender-M	0.986	2.011	2	281	0.136
Gender-F			2	281	
Rhythm-AF	0.997	0.432	2	281	0.650
Rhythm-1st AVB	0.995	0.646	2	281	0.525
Rhythm-SR	0.988	1.711	2	281	0.183
Rhythm-SA	0.991	1.301	2	281	0.274
Rhythm-FAST AF	0.995	0.646	2	281	0.525
Rhythm-S tachy	0.991	1.301	2	281	0.274
Rhythm-slow AF	0.985	2.204	2	281	0.112
Rhythm-BBB	0.985	2.204	2	281	0.112
Rhythm-S brady	0.974	3.823	2	281	0.023
Rhythm-LBBB			2	281	
Rhythm-Pacing R	0.974	3.823	2	281	0.023
Renal Function-Normal	0.714	56.268	2	281	< 0.0001
Renal Function-Abnormal			2	281	
Category-MOD	0.965	5.104	2	281	0.007
Category-NORMAL			2	281	
Category-MILD	0.880	19.221	2	281	< 0.0001
Category-SEVERE	0.883	18.557	2	281	< 0.0001

Plots of component 2 versus component 1 [Figure 19a] revealed clear 'clusterings' (separations) between the three treatment group status classifications (NAV, MPAV and TPAV groups). In particular, the MPAV group of patients had predominantly negative Factor 1 (F1) values, whereas the NAV and TPAV group participants predominantly had positive F1 values. For F2, the majority of the TPAV group patients had positive values for this parameter, whereas most of the NAV classification patients had negative values. Hence, this plot of the F2 versus F1 values for each of the observations demonstrates at least some level of discrimination between the group classifications.

Subsequently, a confusion matrix which summarises a reclassification of the observations was obtained, and this demonstrated that the percentage of correctly-classified observations was equivalent to 72.55, 34.55 and 97.70% for the MPAV, NAV and TPAV patient group classifications respectively [Table 5(a)]. Hence, only the TPAV group could be classified with any degree of near certainty.

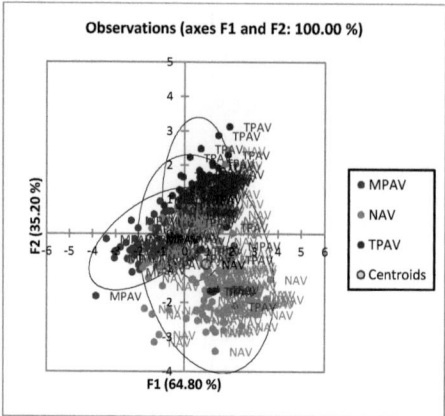

Figure 20(a): Plot of Factor 2 versus Factor 1 for the observations incorporated into the Discriminatory Analysis (DA) model performed on the experimental dataset (missing values were excluded and not estimated). Clearly, there is at least some discrimination achieved between the NAV, MPAV and TPAV groups.

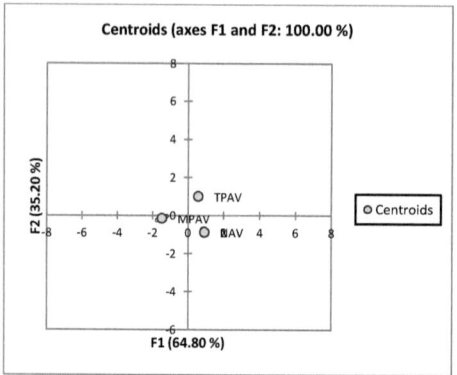

Figure 20 (b) Position of the NAV, MPAV and TPAV group centroids in the plot of Factor 2 versus Factor 1 (corresponding to Figure 3).

Furthermore, predictions for a cross-validation process was then computed [Table 5(b)]; this cross-validation process allowed a determination of the predicted patient group classification for a given observation if first removed from the estimation sample. These predicted classifications gave correctly-classified obsevations of 58.82, 31.51 and 96.55% for the MPAV, NAV and TPAV patient group classifications respectively, i.e., only the TPAV group patients could be correctly predicted with any degree of near certainty. Clearly, for a dataset containing TPAV group patients, only two of the NAV, and one of the MPAV groups of patients were miss-classified.

Table 5(a) Confusion matrix for the estimation sample:

from \ to	MPAV	NAV	TPAV	Total	% correct
MPAV	68.67973856	0	25.9869281	94.66667	72.55%
NAV	3.242009132	32.42009132	59.00456621	94.66667	34.25%
TPAV	1.088122605	1.088122605	92.49042146	94.66667	97.70%
Total	73.0098703	33.50821393	177.4819158	284	68.17%

Table 5(b)

Confusion matrix for the cross-validation results:

from \ to	MPAV	NAV	TPAV	Total	% correct
MPAV	55.68627451	3.712418301	35.26797386	94.66667	58.82%
NAV	3.890410959	29.82648402	60.94977169	94.66667	31.51%
TPAV	1.088122605	2.176245211	91.40229885	94.66667	96.55%
Total	60.66480807	35.71514753	187.6200444	284	62.29%

CHAPTER FIVE

CONCLUSSION AND

REFERENCES

5.1 CONCLUSSION:

In summary, several studies established that medical therapies may have a potential role in reducing the effect of the underlying factors of aortic stenosis progression, in patients in the early stages of this disease process, to slow the progression of severe aortic stenosis and to delay the timing of the need for surgery. However, they show that, the definite AVS cure is aortic valve replacements (AVR) with consideration of high risk patients, such as older people. According to the results of this study, aortic stenosis severity is evaluated on the degree of valve obstruction or narrowing and several other elevated underlying causal factors. The standard parameters are used clinically, for example; the velocity of blood flow through the narrowed aortic valve, the mean pressure gradient between the LV and the aorta, and the cross-sectional area of valve opening. Also, the present study, established that, there are a significant contribution between some of the variable factors and aortic valve stenosis and utilising these decisive variable factors, includes; variables age, maximum velocity, maximum gradient, mean gradient, HDL- Cholesterol and abnormal renal function. Subsequently, among the three groups of patients confusion matrix which summarises a reclassification of the observations was obtained, and thus demonstrated that the percentage of correctly-classified observations was equivalent to 72.55, 34.55 and 97.70% for the MPAV, NAV and TPAV patient group classifications respectively. Hence, only the TPAV group could be classified with any degree of near certainty.

5.2 References:

1. Ashikhmina EA, Schaff HV, Dearani JA, Sundt TM, 3rd, Suri RM, Park SJ, Burkhart HM, Li Z, Daly RC. Aortic valve replacement in the elderly: Determinants of late outcome. Circulation. 2011.

2. Avci I A, Ozcan A, Altyal B, Cavusoglu F. The problem encountered by midwives during breast cancer self-examination training, European Journal of Oncology Nursing. (2008) Vol 12: 329-333.

3. Avdoshin V P, Andriukhin V I, The Russian Radiology and Nuclear Medicine Scientific Center (2005), received the All-Russian Scientific and Practical Conference, Condition and Development of the Russian Federation Mammalogical Service. Radiometric investigation during physiotherapy of chronic adnexitis" Clinical Trial Protocols, Microwave Radiometry in Gynecology,OMan y 2005.

4. Bach DS, Cimino N, Deeb GM. Unoperated patients with severe aortic stenosis. J Am Coll Cardiol. 2007;50:2018-2019.

5. Baglin A, Oldendorf M, Moshage W, Severe valvular heart disease in patients on chronic dialysis, Ann Med Interne (Paris) 1997;148:521–526.

6. Baumgartner H, Hung J, Bermejo J, Chambers JB, Evangelista A, Griffin BP, Iung B, Otto CM, Pellikka PA, Quinones M. Echocardiographic assessment of valve stenosis: Eae/ase recommendations for clinical practice. J Am Soc Echocardiogr. 2009;22:1-23; quiz 101-102.

7. Becher H, ESSENTIAL ECHOCARDIOGRAPH, (2008), page 1-10, 95-110.

8. Bielefeld L , MD, Gerckens U, Schuler G, MD, Bonan R, MD, Kovac J, MD, Patrick W S, MD, Labinaz M, MD, Heijer P D, MD, 2-year follow-up of patients undergoing transcatheter aortic valve implantation using a self-expanding valve prosthesis", Journal of the American College of Cardiology,16,1650-1657,19/04/2011.

9. Bonow R, Braunwald E. Valvular Heart Disease. In: Zipes D, Libby P, Bonow R, Braunwald E, eds. Braunwald's Heart Disease. A textbook of cardiovascular medicine. Philadelphia: Elsevier Saunders, 2005:1553-1632.

10. Bonow RO, Carabello BA, Chatterjee K, de Leon AC, Jr., Faxon DP, Freed MD, Gaasch WH, Lytle BW, Nishimura RA, O'Gara PT, O'Rourke RA, Otto CM, Shah PM, Shanewise JS. 2008 focused update incorporated into the acc/aha 2006 guidelines for the management of patients with valvular heart disease: A report of the american college of cardiology/american heart association task force on practice guidelines (writing committee to revise the 1998 guidelines for the management of patients with valvular heart disease): Endorsed by the society of cardiovascular anesthesiologists, society for cardiovascular angiography and interventions, and society of thoracic surgeons. Circulation. 2008;118:e523-661.

11. Braun J, MD, Oldendorf M MD, Moshage W MD, Electron beam computed tomography in the evaluation of cardiac calcification in chronic dialysis patients, Am J Kidney Dis 1996; 27: 394–401.

12. Bridgewater B, Kinsman R, Walton P, Gummert J and Kappetein AP. The 4th european association for cardio-thoracic surgery adult cardiac surgery database report. Interact Cardiovasc Thorac Surg. 2011;12:4-5

13. Busko M, Echo Predicts Mortality in Aortic Stenosis, Medscape Medical News, American Society of Echocardiography (ASE) 22nd Annual Secientific Sessions, June 11-14,2011 Canada.

14. Cheitlin D M, Armstrong F W. Aurigemma G P, Bierman G A, Davis J L, Douglas P S, Faxon D P, ACC/AHA/ASE, guideline update for the clinical application of echocardiograph, summary article, JOURNAL of the AMERICAN COLLEGE of CARDIOLOGY, J Am Coll Cardiol, 2003; 42:954-970,doi:10.1016/S0735-1097(03)01065-9

15. Chockalingam A, Venkatesan S, Subramaniam T, Jagannathan V, Elangovan S, Alagesan R, Gnanavelu G, Dorairajan S, Krishna BP and Chockalingam V(2004). Safety and efficacy of angiotensin-converting enzyme inhibitors in symptomatic severe aortic stenosis:

Symptomatic cardiac obstruction-pilot study of enalapril in aortic stenosis (scope-as). Am Heart J. 2004;147:E19.

16. Christopher W B, Images in Congenital Cardiac Disease, Unicusp aortic valve, University of Texas Southwestern Children's Medical Centre at Dallas, Dallas, Texas, United States of America, Cardiology in the Young (2010), 20, 557–558, 10.1017/S1047951110000612, Cambridge University Press, 2010, Keywords: Unicommisural aortic valve; aortic valve repair, Received: 9 July 2009; Accepted: 14 March 2010; First published online: 12 July 2010.

17. Cohen G, Zagorski B, Christakis GT, Joyner CD, Vincent J, Sever J, Harbi S, Feder-Elituv R, Moussa F, Goldman BS, Fremes SE. Are stentless valves hemodynamically superior to stented valves? Long-term follow-up of a randomized trial comparing carpentier-edwards pericardial valve with the toronto stentless porcine valve. J Thorac Cardiovasc Surg. 2010;139:848-859.

18. Dare AJ, Veinot JP, Edwards WD, Tazelaar HD, Schaff HV. New observations on the etiology of aortic valve disease: a surgical pathologic study of 236 cases from 1990. Hum Pathol 1993;24:1330-8.

19. Dehghani M, Sharpe L, Nicholas M K, Modification of attentional biases in chronic pain patients: a preliminary study. European Journal of Pain, Vol 8, 585–594.

20. Desai PA, Tafreshi J and Pai RG (2011). Beta-blocker therapy for valvular disorders. J Heart Valve Dis.;20:241-253

21. Desmond J G, Cowan C, and McLenachan J M. Cardiology. 8th ed. Edinburgh: Elsevier Saunders, 2005, page 38,39,72,253-259

22. Eichhorn P, Grimm J, Koch R, Hess O, Carroll J, Krayenbuehl HP. Left ventricular relaxation in patients with left ventricular Myocardial oxygen consumption in aortic valve disease with and without left ventricular dysfunction.Br Heart J. 1992 February; 67(2): 161–169. PMCID: PMC1024747.

23. El-Hamamsy I, Eryigit Z, Stevens LM, Sarang Z, George R, Clark L, Melina G, Takkenberg JJ, Yacoub MH. Long-term outcomes after autograft versus homograft aortic root replacement in adults with aortic valve disease: A randomised controlled trial. Lancet. 2010;376:524-531.

24. Ennezat P V, Marechaux S, Iung B, Chauvel C, LeJemteT H, Pibarot P , Exercise testing and exercise stress echocardiography in asymptomatic aortic valve stenosis, Heart 2009;Published Online First: 23 September 2008, 95: 877-884.

25. Eroglu AG, Babaoglu K , Oztunc F , Saltık L and Demir T, Echocardiographic Follow-Up of Congenital Aortic Valvular Stenosi, Pediatric Cardiology , Received 11 January 2006 / Accepted: 18 July 2006 ,Pediatr Cardiol (2006) 27: 713–719, DOI 10.1007/s00246-006-1321-4.

26. Fournier L S, Dynamic optical breast imaging: A novel technique to detect and characterize tumor vessel. European Journal of Radiology.2008, Vol 26: 256-263.

27. Garcia D, Pibarot P, Kadem L, Durand LG. Respective impacts of aortic stenosis and systemic hypertension on left ventricular hypertrophy. J Biomech. 2007;40:972-980

28. Gersony WM. Natural history of discrete subvalvar aortic stenosis: Management implications. J Am Coll Cardiol. 2001;38:843-845 .

29. Greenbaum RA, Ho SY, Gibson DG, Becker AE, Anderson RH. Left ventricular fibre architecture in man. Br Heart J. 1981;45:248-263.

30. Hammermeister K, Sethi GK, Henderson WG, Grover FL, Oprian C, Rahimtoola SH. Outcomes 15 years after valve replacement with a mechanical versus a bioprosthetic valve: Final report of the veterans affairs randomized trial. J Am Coll Cardiol. 2000;36:1152-1158.

31. Henein MY and Owen A (2010). Statins moderate coronary stenoses but not coronary calcification: Results from meta-analyses. Int J Cardiol.

32. Henein MY, O'Sullivan C, Sutton GC, Gibson DG and Coats AJ, (1997). Stress-induced left ventricular outflow tract obstruction: A potential cause of dyspnea in the elderly.

33. Cardiac Department, Royal Brompton Hospital, London, England, United Kingdom. m.henein@rbh.nthames.nhs.uk. 1997 Nov 1;30(5):1301-7.

34. Hess OM, Villari B, Krayenbuehl HP. Diastolic dysfunction in aortic stenosis. Circulation. 1993;87:IV73-76.

35. Hung J MD, Lang R, MD, Flachskampf F, MD, Shernan S K, MD, McCulloch M L, RDCS, Adams D B, RDCS, Thomas J MD, Vannan M, MD, 3D Echocardiography: A Review of the Current Status and Future Directions, Journal of the American Society of Echocardiography, March 2007, volume 20, number 3, 213-233.

36. Iung B and Vahanian A. Epidemiology of valvular heart disease in the adult. Nat Rev Cardiol. 2011;8:162-172.

37. Iung B, Cachier A, Baron G, Messika-Zeitoun D, Delahaye F, Tornos P, Gohlke-Barwolf C, Boersma E, Ravaud P, Vahanian A. Decision-making in elderly patients with severe aortic stenosis: Why are so many denied surgery? Eur Heart J. 2005;26:2714-2720.

38. Joanna S. Cowell, B.M., David E. Newby, M.D., Robin J. Prescott, Ph.D., Peter Bloomfield, M.D., John Reid, M.B., Ch.B., David B. Northridge, M.D., and Nicholas A.

39. Boon, M.D., A Randomized Trial of Intensive Lipid-Lowering Therapy in Calcific Aortic Stenosis for the Scottish Aortic Stenosis and Lipid Lowering Trial, Impact on Regression (SALTIRE) Investigators N Engl J Med 2005; 352:2389-2397June 9, 2005.

40. Kolh P, Kerzmann A, Honore C, Comte L, Limet R. Aortic valve surgery in octogenarians: Predictive factors for operative and long-term results. Eur J Cardiothorac Surg. 2007;31:600-606.

41. Krayenbuehl HP, Hess OM, Ritter M, Monrad ES, Hoppeler H. Left ventricular systolic function in aortic stenosis. Eur Heart J. 1988;9 Suppl E:19-23.

42. Kunadian B, Vijayalakshmi K, Thornley AR, de Belder MA, Hunter S, Kendall S, Graham R, Stewart M, Thambyrajah J, Dunning J. Meta-analysis of valve hemodynamics and left ventricular mass regression for stentless versus stented aortic valves. Ann Thorac Surg. 2007;84:73-78.

43. Kvidal P, Bergstrom R, Horte LG and Stahle E, (2000). Observed and relative survival after aortic valve replacement. J Am Coll Cardiol;35:747-756

44. Kupari M, Turto H, Lommi J. Left ventricular hypertrophy in aortic valve stenosis: Preventive or promotive of systolic dysfunction and heart failure? Eur Heart J. 2005;26:1790-1796.

45. Leon MB, Smith CR, Mack M, Miller DC, Moses JW, Svensson LG, Tuzcu EM, Webb JG, Fontana GP, Makkar RR, Brown DL, Block PC, Guyton RA, Pichard AD, Bavaria JE, Herrmann HC, Douglas PS, Petersen JL, Akin JJ, Anderson WN and Wang D,

46. Transcatheter aortic-valve for aortic stenosis in implantation patients who cannot undergo surgery. Columbia University Medical Center/New York–Presbyterian Hospital, New York, NY 10032, USA. ml2398@columbia.edu,the New England Journal of Medicine, 2010 Oct 21; 363(17):1597-607. Epub 2010 Sep 22.

47. Leopoldo P I, Zamorano J, Yglesia R P, Cioccarelli S, Almería C , Rodrigo J L , Aubele A L, Herrera D, Mataix L, Carlos V S, Quantification of Aortic Valve Area Using Three-Dimensional Echocardiograph, Revista Espanola de Cardiología. 2008; 61: 494-500. - Vol.61 Num 05 DOI: 10.1016/S1885-5857(08) 60164-4.

48. Lindroos M, Kupari M, Valvanne J, Strandberg T, Heikkila J and Tilvis R. Factors associated with calcific aortic valve degeneration in the elderly. Eur Heart J. 1994;15:865-870.

49. Maher E R, Young G, Smyth-Walsh B, Sara Pugh J R, Calcific aortic Stenosis, A complication of chronic uraemia. Nephron 1987; 47:119–122.

50. Melina G, Mitchell A, Amrani M, Khaghani A, Yacoub MH. Transvalvular velocities after full aortic root replacement: Results from a prospective randomized trial between the

homograft and the medtronic freestyle bioprosthesis. J Heart Valve Dis. 2002;11:54-58; discussion 58-59.

51. Morgan L. Brown, MD, Patricia A. Pellikka, MD, Hartzell V. Schaff, MD, Christopher G. Scott, MS, Charles J. Mullany, MD, Thoralf M MD, Dearani J A, MD, Richard C. D, MD, Thomas A. Orszulak, MD, The benefits of early valve replacement in asymptomatic patients with severe aortic stenosis, The Journal of thorathic and cardiovascular surgery 308-315, 02/ 2008.

52. Nkomo VT, Gardin JM, Skelton TN, Gottdiener JS, Scott CG and Enriquez-Sarano M. Burden of valvular heart diseases: A population-based study. Lancet. 2006;368:1005-1011.

53. Oh JK, Taliercio CP, Holmes DR, Jr., Reeder GS, Bailey KR, Seward JB, Tajik AJ. Prediction of the severity of aortic stenosis by doppler aortic valve area determination: Prospective doppler-catheterization correlation in 100 patients. J Am Coll Cardiol. 1988;11:1227-1234.

54. Osler W, The bicuspid condition of the aortic valves, Transactions of the Association of American Physicians (2000). 1886; 1: 185–92.

55. Perez de Arenaza D, Lees B, Flather M, Nugara F, Husebye T, Jasinski M, Cisowski M, Khan M, Henein M, Gaer J, Guvendik L, Bochenek A, Wos S, Lie M, Van Nooten G, Pennell D, Pepper J. Randomized comparison of stentless versus stented valves for aortic stenosis: Effects on left ventricular mass. Circulation. 2005;112:2696-2702.

56. Perkovic V, Bakri K, Goldsmith D.J.A, Accelerated Progression of Calcific Aortic Stenosis in Dialysis Patients. Nephron Clin Pract , 2003;94:c40-c45 (DOI: 10.1159/000071280.

57. Rahimtoola SH. Valvular heart disease: A perspective on the asymptomatic patient with severe valvular aortic stenosis. Eur Heart J. 2008;29:1783-1790.

58. Raine A, Acquired aortic stenosis in dialysis Patients, Nephron, 1994; 68:159168.

59. Rajamannan NM, Bonow RO and Rahimtoola SH. Calcific aortic stenosis: An update. Nat Clin Pract Cardiovasc Med. 2007;4:254-262

60. Rob B, Gunning M and Nolan J, Essential cardiac catheterization, London: Hodder Arnold, 2007. Page et al (2007). "2-35,249-273.

61. Roberts WC. The structure of the aortic valve in clinically isolated aortic stenosis: An autopsy study of 162 patients over 15 years of age. Circulation. 1970;42:91-97.

62. Rosenhek R, M.D., Binder T, M.D., Porenta G, M.D., Lang I, M.D., Christ G, M.D., Schemper M, Ph.D., Maurer G, M.D., and Baumgartner H, M.D. Predictors of Outcome in Severe, Asymptomatic Aortic Stenosis, N Engl J Med 2000; 343:611-617August 31, 2000.

63. Rossebo AB, Pedersen TR, Boman K, Brudi P, Chambers JB, Egstrup K, Gerdts E, Gohlke-Barwolf C, Holme I, Kesaniemi YA, Malbecq W, Nienaber CA, Ray S, Skjaerpe T, Wachtell K and Willenheimer R, (2008). Intensive lipid lowering with simvastatin and ezetimibe in aortic stenosis. N Engl J Med.;359:1343-1356.

64. Silverman D, Qualitative research: Reliability and validity in research based on naturally occurring social interaction, .2nd ed. Sage publication. P 282-287.

65. Silverman D, Qualitative research: Reliability and validity in research based on naturally occurring social interaction, .2nd ed,(2004) Sage publication. P 282-287 .

66. Somers P, Knaapen M, Mistiaen W. Histopathology of calcific aortic valve stenosis. Acta Cardiol. 2006;61:557-562.

67. Spence. S.H. Cognitive-behavior therapy in the management of chronic, occupational pain of the upper limbs. Behaviour Research and Therapy. (1989) Vol 27. 4: 435-446.

68. Stewart BF, Siscovick D, Lind BK, Gardin JM, Gottdiener JS, Smith VE, Kitzman DW and Otto CM. Clinical factors associated with calcific aortic valve disease. Cardiovascular health study. J Am Coll Cardiol. 1997;29:630-634.

69. Takeda S, Rimington H, Smeeton N, Chambers J. Long axis excursion in aortic stenosis. Heart. 2001;86:52-56.

70. Tarantini G, Buja P, Scognamiglio R, Razzolini R, Gerosa G, Isabella G, Ramondo A, Iliceto S. Aortic valve replacement in severe aortic stenosis with left ventricular dysfunction: Determinants of cardiac mortality and ventricular function recovery. Eur J Cardiothorac Surg. 2003;24:879-885.

71. Teo KK, Corsi DJ, Tam JW, Dumesnil JG and Chan KL (2011). Lipid lowering on progression of mild to moderate aortic stenosis: Meta-analysis of the randomized placebo-controlled clinical trials on 2344 patients.

72. Thomson HL, O'Brien MF, Almeida AA, Tesar PJ, Davison MB, Burstow DJ. Haemodynamics and left ventricular mass regression: A comparison of the stentless, stented and mechanical aortic valve replacement. Eur J Cardiothorac Surg. 1998;13:572-575.

73. Toutouzas K, Syneros A, Drakopoulou M and Grassos C, Abstract 15140: Microwave Radiometry for the Detection of Local Inflammatory Activation in Atherosclerotic Plaques": A New Non-Invasive Method. Circulation. 2010; 122: A15140.

74. Vahanian A, Baumgartner H, Bax J, Butchart E, Dion R, Filippatos G, Frank A, Hall R, Iung B, Kasprzak J D, European Society of Cardiology European Heart Journal, Guidelines on the management of valvular heart disease, European Society of Cardiology European Heart Journal 2007; 28: 230-268.

75. Villa E, Troise G, Cirillo M, Brunelli F, Tomba MD, Mhagna Z, Tasca G, Quaini E. Factors affecting left ventricular remodeling after valve replacement for aortic stenosis. An overview. Cardiovasc Ultrasound. 2006;4:25.

76. Wanger S G, Marriott's Practical Electrocardiography, 11th edition (2008) chapter 1, 1-17.

77. Zaca V, Ballo P, Galderisi M, Mondillo S. Echocardiography in the assessment of left ventricular longitudinal systolic function: Current methodology and clinical applications. Heart Fail Rev. 2010;15:23-37.

78. Zoghbi WA, Chambers JB, Dumesnil JG, Foster E, Gottdiener JS, Grayburn PA, Khandheria BK, Levine RA, Marx GR, Miller FA, Jr., Nakatani S, Quinones MA, Rakowski H, Rodriguez LL, Swaminathan M, Waggoner AD, Weissman NJ and Zabalgoitia M.

Recommendations for evaluation of prosthetic valves with echocardiography and doppler ultrasound: A report from the american society of echocardiography's guidelines and standards committee and the task force on prosthetic valves, developed in conjunction with the american college of cardiology cardiovascular imaging committee, cardiac imaging committee of the american heart association, the european association of echocardiography, a registered branch of the european society of cardiology, the japanese society of echocardiography and the canadian society of echocardiography, endorsed by the american college of cardiology foundation, american heart association, european association of echocardiography, a registered branch of the european society of cardiology, the japanese society of echocardiography, and canadian society of echocardiography. J Am Soc Echocardiogr. 2009;22:975-1014; quiz 1082-1014

79. Skowasch D, Steinmetz M, Nickenig, G and Bauriedel G , (2006), Is the degeneration of aortic valve bioprostheses similar to that of native aortic valves? Insights into valvular pathology, Source: EXPERT REVIEW OF MEDICAL DEVICES Volume: 3 Issue: 4Pages: 453-462 DOI: 10.1586/17434440.3.4.453 Published: JUL 2006

80. Mao M, El Ters M, Mankad S, Mira K, Park S, and Qian Q, (2011). Prosthetic Aortic Valve Stenosis in End-Stage Renal Failure. 1Division of Nephrology and Hypertension, Department of Medicine, Mayo Clinic, Rochester, MN 55902, USA2Division of Cardiology, Department of Medicine, Mayo Clinic, Rochester, MN 55902, USA3Department of Surgery, Mayo Clinic, Rochester, MN 55902, USA. Received 2 February 2011; Accepted 18 March 2011

81. Jacob D P, Partho S P and Bijoy K K, (2008), Role of echocardiography in the diagnosis and management of asymptomatic severe aortic stenosis. Source: Expert review of cardiovascular therapy Volume: 6 Issue: 2 Pages: 223-33 DOI: 10.1586/14779072.6.2.223 Published: 2008-Feb.

82. Ohashi K L, Culkar J, Riebman J B, Estes M, Constantz B R and Yoganathan A P (2004). Hemodynamic Characterization of Calcified Stenotic, Human Aortic Valves Before and After Treatment with abNovel Aortic Valve Repair System. 1Corazón Technologies, Inc., Menlo Park, CA, 2Santa Clara Valley Medical Center, San Jose, CA, 3Department of Mechanical Engineering, Stanford University, Stanford, CA, 4Wallace H. Coulter,

Department of Biomedical Engineering, Georgia Institute of Technology and Emory University, Atlanta, GA, USA. The Journal of Heart Valve Disease 2004;13:582-592.

83. Stout K K and Otto C M, (2007). Indications for Aortic Valve Replacement in Aortic Stenosis. Journal of Intensive Care Medicine. http://jic.sagepub.com/content/22/1/14. The online version of this article can be found at: DOI: 10.1177/0885066606295298. J Intensive Care Med 2007 22: 14. Published by:http://www.sagepublications.com.

84. Soyer R, Bouchart F, Bessou JP), Redonnet M, MoutonSchleifer D, Derumeaux G, Arrignon J and Letac B, (1996) Aortic valve replacement after aortic valvuloplasty for calcified aortic stenosis Source: EUROPEAN JOURNAL OF CARDIO-THORACIC SURGERY Volume: 10 Issue: 11 Pages: 977-982 DOI: 10.1016/S1010-7940(96)80400-3 Published: NOV 1996

85. Rajamannan NM, (2010), Mechanisms of aortic valve calcification: the LDL-density-radius theory: a translation from cell signaling to physiology Source: AMERICAN JOURNAL OF PHYSIOLOGY-HEART AND CIRCULATORY PHYSIOLOGY Volume: 298 Issue: 1 Pages: H5-H15 DOI: 10.1152/ajpheart.00824.2009 Published: JAN 2010. Times Cited: 8 (from Web of Science).

86. Jacob D P, Partho S P and Bijoy K K, (2008), Role of echocardiography in the diagnosis and management of asymptomatic severe aortic stenosis. Source: Expert review of cardiovascular therapy Volume: 6 Issue: 2 Pages: 223-33 DOI: 10.1586/14779072.6.2.223 Published: 2008-Feb.

87. Sun J, and Li H, (2012) Financial distress prediction using support vector machines: Ensemble vs. individual, School of Economics and Management, Zhejiang Normal University, Jinhua City, Zhejiang Province 321004, China

88. Otto C M,(2010) Calciofic Aortic Valve Disease: New Concepts, Semin Thoracic Surg 22:276-284@2010 Elsevier inc. All right reserved.

89. Baumgartner H, Hung J, Bermejo J, Chambers J B, Evangelista A, Griffin B P, Iung B, Otto C M, Pellikka P A and Quin¨ones M, (2009), Echocardiographic assessment of valve stenosis: EAE/ASErecommendations for clinical practice. 1University of Muenster,

Muenster, Germany; 2Massachusetts General Hospital, Boston, MA, USA; 3Hospital General Universitario Gregorio Maran~o´n, Barcelona, Spain; 4Huy's and St. Thomas' Hospital, London, United Kingdom; 5Hospital Vall D'Hebron, Barcelona, Spain; 6Cleveland Clinic, Cleveland, OH, USA; 7Paris VII Denis Diderot University, Paris, France; 8University of Washington, Seattle, WA, USA; 9Mayo Clinic, Rochester, MN, USA; and 10The Methodist Hospital, Houston, TX, USA European Journal of Echocardiography (2009) 10, 1–25 doi:10.1093/ejechocard/jen303

90. Osrane k, Pilip A, PateP R, Molisse T, Tunick P A and , Kronzon I, (2008), Amounts of Aortic Atherosclerosis in Patients With Aortic Stenosis as Determined by Transesophageal Echocardiography, The American Journal of Cardiology, Department of Noninvasive Cardiology, New York University School of Medicine, New York, New Yorhttp://dx.doi.org/10.1016/j.amjcard.2008.11.026, How to Cite or Link Using DOI, Permissions & Reprints.

91. Rosenhek R, Binder T, Porenta G, Lang I, Christ G, Schemper M, Maurer G, Baumgartner H.(2000),Predictors of outcome in severe, asymptomatic aortic stenosis. Department of Cardiology, Vienna General Hospital, and Ludwig Boltzmann Institute for Cardiovascular Research, Austria, N Engl J Med. 2000 Aug 31;343(9):611-7

92. ACC/AHA 2006 Guidelines for the Management of Patients With Valvular Heart Disease, A Report of the American College of Cardiology/American Heart Association Task Force on Practice Guidelines (Writing Committee to Revise the 1998 Guidelines for the Management of Patients With Valvular Heart Disease) Developed in Collaboration With the Society of Cardiovascular Anesthesiologists Endorsed by the Society for Cardiovascular Angiography and Interventions and the Society of Thoracic Surgeons . Journal of the American College of Cardiology , Volume 48 , Issue 3 , Pages e1 - e148

93. Pibarot P and Dumesnil J G, 92011), Improving Assessment of Aortic Stenosis, Québec Heart and Lung Institute, Department of Medicine, Laval University, Québec, Québec, Canadahttp://dx.doi.org.ezproxy.liv.ac.uk/10.1016/j.jacc.2011.11.078, How to Cite or Link Using DOIPermissions & Reprints, Journal of the American College of CardiologyVolume 60, Issue 3, 17 July 2012, Pages 169–180

94. Francis J, (2008), Aortic stenosis: Echocardiogram in parasternal short axis view Posted on October 30, 2008, Cardiophile MD.

95. O'Gara T, Robert A. O'Rourke, Catherine M. Otto P, Shah M. and. Shanewise J S, Faxon F, Gaasch W H, Lytle B W, Nishimura R A, Bonow P R, Carabello B A, Chatterjee K, de Leon A C and David Jr P,(2006), Cardiovascular Angiography and Interventions and the Society of Thoracic Surgeons the Society of Cardiovascular Anesthesiologists: Endorsed by the Society for Management of Patients With Valvular Heart Disease): Developed in Collaboration With on Practice Guidelines (Writing Committee to Revise the 1998 Guidelines for the A Report of the American College of Cardiology/American Heart Association Task Force ACC/AHA 2006 Guidelines for the Management of Patients With Valvular Heart Disease : Print ISSN: 0009-7322. Online ISSN: 1524-4539 Copyright © 2006 American Heart Association, Inc. All rights reserved. Circulation is published by the American Heart Association, 7272 Greenville Avenue, Dallas, TX 75231

96. Stevens LA, Coresh J, Greene T, Levey AS. Assessing kidney function--measured and estimated glomerular filtration rate. N Engl J Med 2006; 354:2473

97. Julian D G, Campbel JC and McLenachan J M, "2005), CARDIOLOGY, EIGHT EDITION, page 85, 234.

98. Becher H, (2008), Essential Echocardiography, John Radcliffe Hospital, Oxford, UK, first published 2008, ISBN 9780443103230, PAGE, 39, 236.

99. Birtcher K K and Ballantyne C M, (2004), Measurement of Cholesterol. 1-From the College of Pharmacy, University of Houston, and the Kelsey-Seybold Clinic (K.K.B.), and the Section of Atherosclerosis and Lipoprotein Research, Department of Medicine, Baylor College of Medicine, and the Center for Cardiovascular Disease Prevention, Methodist DeBakey Heart Center (C.M.B.), Houston, Tex. 2- Correspondence to Christie M. Ballantyne, MD, Baylor College of Medicine, 656 Fannin, M.S. A-601, Houston, TX 77030. E-mail cmb@bcm.tmc.edu. Circulation. 2004; 110: e296-e297 doi: 10.1161/01.CIR.0000141564.89465.4E

100.Nosir Y. F M , Paolo FM, Vletter W B Boersma E , Salustri , Tjoa Postma T, Reijs A E M, Ten Cate F and Roelandt J R, (1996), A Comparison With Radionuclide Angiography, Accurate Measurement of Left Ventricular Ejection Fraction by Three-dimensional Echocardiography, 1-the Thoraxcenter, Division of Cardiology, and Department of Nuclear Medicine, University Hospital Rotterdam-Dijkzigt, and Erasmus University, Rotterdam, Netherlands. 2-mCorrespondence to Paolo M. Fioretti, MD, Thoraxcenter, Ba 300, Dr Molewaterplein 40, 3015 GD Rotterdam, Netherlands.

101.Bach D S, Schmitz , Dohmen G , Aaronson K D, Steinseifer U and, Kleine , (2011), In vitro assessment of prosthesis type and pressure recovery characteristics: Doppler echocardiography overestimation of bileaflet mechanical and bioprosthetic aortic valve gradients, Division of Cardiovascular Medicine, Department of Internal Medicine, University of Michigan, Ann Arbor, Mich, b Department of Cardiovascular Engineering, Helmholtz Institute, RWTH Aachen University, Aachen, Germany, c Department of Thoracic and Cardiovascular Surgery, University Hospital Aachen, Aachen, Germand Department of Thoracic and Cardiovascular Surgery, J. W. Goethe University, Frankfurt am Main, Germanhttp://dx.doi.org.ezproxy.liv.ac.uk/10.1016/j.jtcvs.2011.12.036, How to Cite or Link Using DOI.Permissions & Reprints Received 21 September 20Revised 18 November 2011

102.Creswell J W, (2012). Educational research: Planning, conducting, and evaluating quantitative and qualitative research. Upper Saddle River, NJ: Prentice Hall.

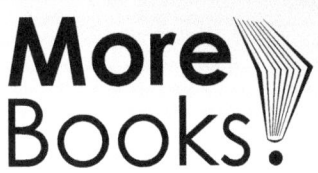
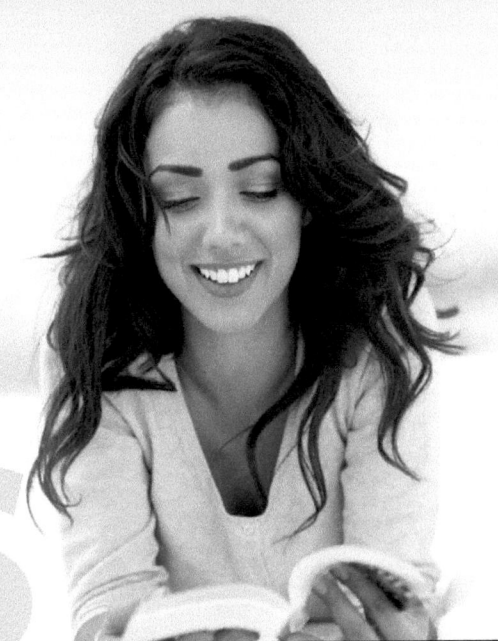

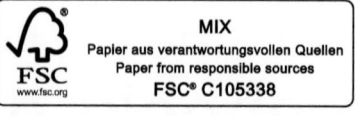

Printed by Books on Demand GmbH, Norderstedt / Germany